Interventional
Pain Management
A Practical Approach

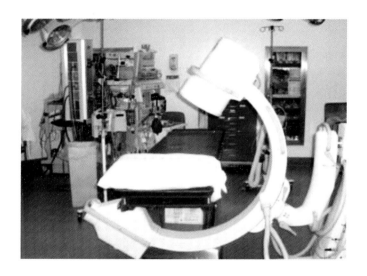

Under the aegis
of
Bombay Hospital Institute of Medical Sciences
and
Pain Management and Research Foundation (India)

Interventional Pain Management

A Practical Approach

Editors

DK Baheti MD
Chief of Anaesthesiology and
Pain Management Clinic
Bombay Hospital Institute of Medical Sciences, Mumbai, India

Sanjay Bakshi MD
Interventional Pain Management
Lenox Hill Hospital, New York, USA
Beth Israel Hospital, New York, USA
Spine and Pain Medicine
899 Park Avenue, NY 10021, USA

Sanjeeva Gupta MD, Dip. NB, FRCA, FIPP
Consultant in Pain Management and Anaesthesia
Bradford Teaching Hospitals NHS Foundation Trust
Department of Anaesthesia, Pain Management and Critical Care,
Field House, Bradford Royal Infirmary, Duckworth Lane,
Bradford, BD9 6RJ, United Kingdom

RP Gehdoo MD, DA
Professor of Anaesthesia,
Tata Memorial Hospital, Parel, Mumbai (India)

JAYPEE BROTHERS MEDICAL PUBLISHERS (P) LTD

New Delhi · Ahmedabad · Bengaluru · Chennai · Hyderabad · Kochi
Kolkata · Lucknow · Mumbai · Nagpur

Published by
Jitendar P Vij
Jaypee Brothers Medical Publishers (P) Ltd
Corporate Office
4838/24 Ansari Road, Daryaganj, **New Delhi** - 110002, India, Phone: +91-11-43574357
Registered Office
B-3 EMCA House, 23/23B Ansari Road, Daryaganj, **New Delhi** - 110 002, India
Phones: +91-11-23272143, +91-11-23272703, +91-11-23282021
+91-11-23245672, Rel: +91-11-32558559, Fax: +91-11-23276490, +91-11-23245683
e-mail: jaypee@jaypeebrothers.com, Visit our website: www.jaypeebrothers.com

Branches

- ❑ 2/B, Akruti Society, Jodhpur Gam Road Satellite
  Ahmedabad 380 015, Phones: +91-79-26926233, Rel: +91-79-32988717
  Fax: +91-79-26927094 e-mail: ahmedabad@jaypeebrothers.com

- ❑ 202 Batavia Chambers, 8 Kumara Krupa Road, Kumara Park East
  Bengaluru 560 001, Phones: +91-80-22285971, +91-80-22382956, 91-80-22372664
  Rel: +91-80-32714073, Fax: +91-80-2228176 e-mail: bangalore@jaypeebrothers.com

- ❑ 282 IIIrd Floor, Khaleel Shirazi Estate, Fountain Plaza, Pantheon Road
  Chennai 600 008, Phones: +91-44-28193265, +91-44-28194897, Rel: +91-44-32972089
  Fax: +91-44-2819323 e-mail: chennai@jaypeebrothers.com

- ❑ 4-2-1067/1-3, 1st Floor, Balaji Building, Ramkote Cross Road,
  Hyderabad 500 095, Phones: +91-40-66610020, +91-40-24758498
  Rel:+91-40-32940929, Fax:+91-40-24758499 e-mail: hyderabad@jaypeebrothers.com

- ❑ No. 41/3098, B & B1, Kuruvi Building, St. Vincent Road
  Kochi 682 018, Kerala, Phones: +91-484-4036109, +91-484-2395739
  +91-484-2395740 e-mail: kochi@jaypeebrothers.com

- ❑ 1-A Indian Mirror Street, Wellington Square
  Kolkata 700 013, Phones: +91-33-22651926, +91-33-22276404
  +91-33-22276415, Rel: +91-33-32901926, Fax: +91-33-22656075
  e-mail: kolkata@jaypeebrothers.com

- ❑ Lekhraj Market III, B-2, Sector-4, Faizabad Road, Indira Nagar
  Lucknow 226 016, Phones: +91-522-3040553, +91-522-3040554
  e-mail: lucknow@jaypeebrothers.com

- ❑ 106 Amit Industrial Estate, 61 Dr SS Rao Road, Near MGM Hospital, Parel
  Mumbai 400 012, Phones: +91-22-24124863, +91-22-24104532,
  Rel: +91-22-32926896, Fax: +91-22-24160828
  e-mail: mumbai@jaypeebrothers.com

- ❑ "KAMALPUSHPA" 38, Reshimbag, Opp. Mohota Science College, Umred Road
  Nagpur 440 009 (MS), Phone: Rel: +91-712-3245220, Fax: +91-712-2704275
  e-mail: nagpur@jaypeebrothers.com

USA Office
1745, Pheasant Run Drive, Maryland Heights (Missouri), MO 63043, USA
Ph: 001-636-6279734
e-mail: jaypee@jaypeebrothers.com, anjulav@jaypeebrothers.com

Interventional Pain Management—A Practical Approach

© 2009, Jaypee Brothers Medical Publishers

First Edition: 2009

ISBN 978-81-8448-319-2

Typeset at JPBMP typesetting unit
Printed at Sanat Printers, Kundli.

Dedicated

to

All Pain Patients

Contributors

Abrahemsen Gerard W, RPA-C
Interventional Pain Management
Lenox Hill Hospital, New York, USA
Beth Israel Hospital, New York, USA
Spine and Pain Medicine
899 Park Avenue, NY 10021, USA
Website-www.spineandpain.com

Baheti DK MD
Chief of Anaesthesiology and
Pain Management Clinic
Bombay Hospital Institute of Medical
Sciences, 12, New Marine Lines
Mumbai-400 020, India
email-drbaheti@rediffmail.com /
dr.baheti@gmail.com
Website-painmanagementindia.com

Bakshi Sanjay MD
Interventional Pain Management
Lenox Hill Hospital, New York, USA
Beth Israel Hospital, New York, USA
Spine and Pain Medicine
899 Park Avenue, NY 10021, USA
email-drbakshi@spineandpain.com
Website-www.spineandpain.com

Boswell Marks V MD, PHD
Professor of Anaesthesiology
Interim Department Chair and Director
of the Messer Racz Pain Center
Department of Anesthesiology, Texas
Tech University Health Sciences Center
3401 4th Street STOP 8182, Lubbock,
Texas 79430

Dalvie Samir MS (ORTH), D ORTH FCPS,
DNBE
Spine Surgeon
Bombay Hospital and Medical
Research Centre, Mumbai 400020
Email:sdalvie@hotmail.com

Das Gautam MD
Director of Pain Clinic,
Daradia: The Pain Clinic
92/2A Bidhannagar Road
Kolkata -700067
India
Email: info@painindia.net
Website: www.painindia.net

Diwan Sudhir MD
Director, Division of Pain Medicine
Director, Pain Medicine Fellowship
Program
New York Presbyterian Hospital
Weill Medical College of Cornell
University
525 East 68th Street, New York
NY 10021, USA
Email-sad2003@med.cornell.edu

Doshi Preeti MD, MDDA [UK], FRCAII [LON]
Consultant Pain Specialist and
Incharge of pain Clinic
Jaslok Hospital and Research Centre
15, Dr G Deshmukh Road
Mumbai-400026, India
Email-preetipd@gmail.com
Website-www.jaslokhospital.net

Doshi Paresh K MS MCH
Incharge, Stereo tactic and Functional
Neurosurgical Program
Jaslok Hospital and Research Centre
15, Dr G Deshmukh Marg
Mumbai - 400016
pareshkd@gmail.com
www.parkinsonsdiseasesurgery.net

Gehdoo RP MD, DA
Professor of Anaesthesia
Tata Memorial Hospital
Parel, Mumbai- 400 012
India
email-rpgk1@rediffmail.com

Gupta Sanjeeva, MD, DIP NB, FRCA, FIPP
Consultant in Pain Management and
Anaesthesia
Bradford Teaching Hospitals NHS
Foundation Trust
Department of Anaesthesia
Pain Management and Critical Care
Field House, Bradford Royal
infirmary, Duckworth Lane,
Bradford, BD9 6RJ, United Kingdom.
Email: SGupta6502@aol.com

Heavner James DVM, PHD
Professor, Department of
Anesthesiology
Texas Tech University Health Sciences
Center
Lubbock, TX
james.heavner@ttuhsc.edu

Jain Jitendra MD
Pain Physician, Spine and Pain Clinic,
Diamond palace, opposite Bandra
Police station, Hill Road, Bnadra west,
Mumbai 400050, Maharashtra, India
Website: www.spineandpain.org

Jain PN MD MNAMS
Professor, Anaesthesiology,
Tata Memorial Hospital
Mumbai 400 012
Email-pnj5@hotmail.com

Jhankaria Bhavin MD
Director, Jhanakaria Imaging Centre
Bhaveshawar Vihar, 383, Sardar VP
Road, Mumbai-400 004

Kothari Kailash MD
Pain Physician, Wockhard Hospital
Mumbai, India
Email-drkothari@yahoo.com

Krishnan Pradeep MBBS
Jhanakaria Imaging Centre
Bhaveshawar Vihar, 383, Sardar VP
Road, Mumbai-400 004

Manchikanti Laxmaiah, MD
Medical Director, Pain Management
Center of Paducah
Associate Clinical Professor
Anesthesiology and Perioperative
Medicine
University of Louisville, Kentucky
2831 Lone Oak Road, Paducah,
KY 42003
E-mail: drm@asipp.org

Mangeshikar Tilottama MD
Consultant Anesthesiologist and
Interventional Pain Physician
Cumballa Hill Hospital, Madhav
Niwas, 8 Laburnum Rd, Gamdevi
Mumbai 400007
Email-tilu@mangeshikar.com
website-
www.totalpainmanagementclinic.com

Pathak Sachin MBBS
Jhanakaria Imaging Centre
Bhaveshawar Vihar, 383, Sardar V.P.
Road, Mumbai-400 004

Patrick F Annello MD
Pain Management Fellow
New York Presbyterian Weill-Cornell
University Medical Center
Email-Annello18setter@hotmail.com

Piparia Vishal DMRD
Jhanakaria Imaging Centre
Bhaveshawar Vihar, 383, Sardar VP
Road, Mumbai-400 004

Rai Sarvendra MBBS
Registrar, Dept. of Neurosurgery.
Jaslok Hospital and Research Centre
15, Dr. G. Deshmukh Marg, Mumbai –
India-400016

Richardson Jonathan MD, FRCA, FRCP, FIPP
Consultant in Pain Management
Bradford Teaching Hospitals NHS
Foundation Trust
Department of Anaesthesia, Pain
Management and Critical Care,
Field House, Bradford Royal infirmary,
Duckworth Lane,
Bradford, BD9 6RJ, United Kingdom.
Email: docjohnnyr@hotmail.com

Bram Harris MD, DABPM
Monmouth Medical Center
Long Branch
NJ, USA

Shah Rinoo V MD
Assistant Professor, Interventional
Pain Management
Department of Anesthesiology
Guthrie Clinic, Sayre, PA
email-rinoo_shah@yahoo.com

Sharma Anil K MD, DABPM
Director of Pain Management
Monmouth Medical Center
Long Branch, NJ USA

Tarcatu Dana MD
Fellow, Pain and Palliative Care
Memorial Sloan-Kettering Cancer
Center, Department of Neurology
1275 York Avenue, NY, NY 10021
tarcatud@mskcc.org

Foreword

Dr. B.K. Goyal

FAMS (IND), FRCP (EDIN), FSCAI, FACC (USA), B.Sc., MB, DTM & H (LIV), FICP, FICC, FICA (NY), FIMSA, MICTD (BER), FCCP (USA), FRSTM (LOND)

INTERVENTIONAL CARDIOLOGIST

Lotus House, Marine Lines, Mumbai 400 020
Tel.: 2203 7777 / 2201 0000

Bom Hos: 2203 2222 • 2206 7676 • Mobile : 98201 54445
Residence : 2367 9999 • Fax : 91-22-2201 0000
e-mail : drbkgoyal@hotmail.com

- **DIRECTOR INTERVENTIONAL CARDIOLOGY & HON. DEAN**
  Bombay Hospital & Medical Research Centre
- **VISITING CARDIOLOGIST**
  Breach Candy Hospital
- **HON. CONSULTANT CARDIOLOGIST**
  Texas Heart Institute, Housecon, Texas, USA
- **AWARDED BY PRESIDENT OF INDIA**
  Padma Vibhushan, Padma Bhushan & Padma Shri
- **EDITOR**
  Journal of American College of Cardiology
  (S.E. Asian Edition)
- **FORMER SHERIFF OF BOMBAY**

Pain is an integral part of the sufferings of human life. One can only realize agony when one suffers from it. Pain especially a chronic one, is not a mere symptom, it itself is a disease. Chronic pain not only disturbs various systems of the body, but also is responsible for emotional disturbances and can lead to loss of working hours.

Pain management is fast growing as superspeciality of anaesthesiology in India. In USA and other western countries pain management is already established as a superspeciality subject.

At Bombay Hospital, Dr DK Baheti, Chief of Anaesthesiology, realized the need for development of pain clinic. He visited Cleveland Clinic and Memorial Sloan-Kettering Cancer Centre for the first hand training.

For the last 17 years he has been successfully managing the Pain Management clinic at Bombay Hospital. During this period he organized international conferences like Global Update on Pain, conducted live demonstrations and hands on cadaver workshops for training young anaesthesiologists at Bombay Hospital.

Interventional pain procedures are important modalities for relief of pain. Dr DK Baheti, along with Dr Sanjay Bakshi (USA), Dr Sanjeeva Gupta (UK), and Dr RP Gehdoo (Mumbai) have joined hands to bring out a comprehensive book on Interventional Pain Management.

I am confident that this book will be very useful as a reference book for the medical students and will also provide practical tips to practicing physicians and young anaesthesiologists whose mission is to relieve humanity from the agony of sufferings.

(Dr B K Goyal)

Preface

Interventional pain management is one of the most important components of managing chronic intractable pain. It is mandatory that interventional procedures need to be performed correctly right from the time of diagnosis to the relief of pain, so as to provide the best possible results.

Many universities in India as well as abroad do not have appropriate pain training program in their curriculum not only at the undergraduate but, also at postgraduate levels. There are very few pain certification programs or pain specialists or pain training facilities across the world.

Even in the countries where such programs exist, there are significant inadequacies and lacunae in teaching of the techniques. Although there are courses run by various organizations, they only incorporate a few common techniques and hence can never be comprehensive.

Many pain physicians are enthusiastic to learn the art of interventional techniques for managing pain, but do not have an access to appropriate reference books. The availability and cost of the books adds to further constraints.

We, the practicing pain physicians, have recognized the problem and realized the need for a book on Interventional Pain Management techniques, which can be both comprehensive and affordable.

It is our sincere attempt to come out with a book on interventional pain procedures due to existing vacuum in this field.

We express our heartfelt gratitude to all the contributors, without whose support this Herculean task would have been impossible.

We have taken utmost care to bring out this book with an international quality at an affordable price.

We sincerely hope that our efforts to come out with this book will benefit the pain physicians as well as the chronic pain patients.

DK Baheti, Sanjay Bakshi
Sanjeeva Gupta, RP Gehdoo

Contents

SECTION - D
Chest and Thorax

SECTION - E
Abdomen and Pelvis

SECTION - F
Spine and Back

SECTION - G
Advanced Pain Management

SECTION - H
What's New in Interventional Pain Management?

SECTION - I
Alternate Therapies

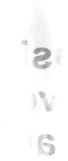

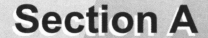

Section A

Basics in Interventional Pain Management

One

Basis of Radiological Imaging

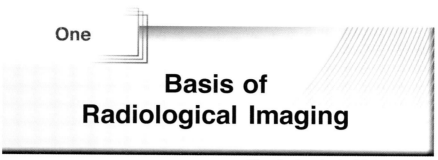

Bhavin Jhankaria, Vishal Piparia

HISTORY

Wilhelm Conrad Roentgen, a German physicist discovered X-rays on November 8, 1895. Roentgen was investigating the behavior of cathode rays (electron) in high energy cathode ray tube. The tube consisted of glass envelope from which most of the air is removed. A short platinum electrode was fitted into each end and when a high voltage discharge was passed through the tube, ionization of remaining gas produced a faint light. Roentgen had enclosed his cathode ray tube in black card board to prevent this light from escaping the tube. On passing a high voltage discharge through the tube, he noticed a faint light glowing on a work bench 3 feet away. Because electrons could not escape the glass envelope.

Roentgen concluded that some unknown type of ray was produced, when the tube was energized. He began placing the tube and the fluorescent screen: a book, a block of wood and a sheet of aluminum. The brightness of the fluorescence differed with each, indicating that the ray penetrated some objects more easily than others. Finally he held his hand between the tube and screen, and the outline of his skeleton appeared.

Till December 28, 1895, he thoroughly experimented and he was awarded the first Nobel Prize for physics in 1901 for discovery of X-rays.

ATOMIC STRUCTURE

In 1987, JJ Thompson discovered a negatively charged particle called as electron. Based on the work of Rutherford and Bohv, a model of atom was made. Thus an atom consists of positively charged nucleus and surrounded by electrons in orbit.

The nucleus consists of mainly protons and neutrons. The proton has positive charge while neutron has zero electrical charge. The no. of protons in the nucleus is called atomic no. (Z). the total no. of protons and neutrons in the nucleus of atom is called as mass number (A) (Fig. 1.1).

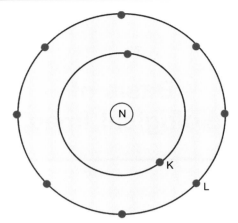

Fig. 1.1: Basic atom

ELECTRON ORBITS AND ENERGY LEVELS

The electrons are negatively charged particles revolving around the nucleus. An electrically neutral atom contains equal no. of protons and neutrons. The electron move in orbit of shells with 2 in 1st orbit, 8 in 2nd and 18 in 3rd and so on. Three orbits are designated as K, L, M, N, and O and so on.

The attractive force between the positively charged nucleus and negatively charged electron is called as binding force. This force is inversely proportional to the square of distance between the nucleus and electron. This attractive force keeps the electron moving in circular path.

To free an electron from an atom, the energy must be raised to zero to a positive value. The energy that an electron in shell needs to rise to zero or a positive value is called as binding energy of the electron. Ex. To free a 'K' electron from tungsten the electron must be given 70 KeV of energy while only 11 KeV is required to free 'L' electron. The binding energy of electron shells varies from one element to other. The electron can jump from one shell to other shells. The electron moving to lower energy shell results in emission of energy.

ELECTROMAGNETIC SPECTRUM

X- rays belong to a group of radiation called electromagnetic radiation. It is the transport of energy through space as combustion of electric and magnetic fields. The electromagnetic radiation is made up of an electric field and a magnetic field that naturally support each other.

The wave concept of Electromagnetic radiation (EM): The EM radiation is propagated through the space in the form of waves. The no. of waves passing a particular point of time is called as frequency. The wavelength of diagnostic X-rays is extremely short and it is expressed in Angstrom Units (A).

The particle concept of EM radiation: Short EM waves like X-rays react with matter, as if they are particles and not waves. These particles are actually discrete bundles of energy and each of these bundles of energy is called "Photon". The actual amount of energy of Photon is calculated by multiplying, it's frequency by a constant.

E= hv
E= photon energy
H= pluck's constant
V= frequency

The unit used to measure the energy of photon is called as electron volt (eV).

PRODUCTION OF X-RAYS

X-ray Tube (Fig. 1.2)

X-rays is produced by energy conversion when a fast moving stream of electrons is suddenly decelerated in the target anode of X-ray tube. The X-ray tube is made of Pyrex glass that encloses a vacuum containing two electrode (diode tube).

The electrons are produced at the cathode end (filament), which are accelerated by a high potential difference towards the anode end (positive/target) where X-rays are produced.

Glass Enclosure

The glass tube encloses two electrodes in vacuum. If gas is present inside the tube, the electrons which are accelerated towards the anode would collide with the gas molecules, loose energy and cause secondary electrons to be ejected from gas molecule by a process of ionization. Thus there is vacuum in

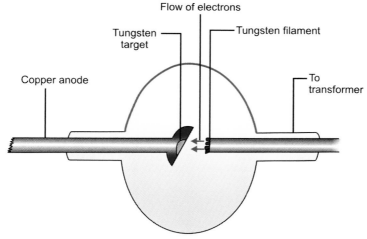

Fig. 1.2: Basic X-ray tube

modern X-ray tube. The connecting wires must be sealed into glass wall of X-ray tube. These are made up of special alloys to prevent the breaking of glass metal seal.

CATHODE

Cathode is a negative terminal of X-ray tube. In addition to this filament, there are connecting wires which supply both the voltage and amperage. The X-ray tube current is measured in milli amperes MA, refers to the no. of electrons flowing per second from cathode to anode. The cathode end, i.e. the filament is made up of tungsten wire 0.2 mm in diameter that is coiled to form a vertical spiral about 0.2 cm in diameter and 1cm or less in length. When this filament is heated, it connects electron by the process of thermion emission. The electron cloud surrounding the filament by thermion emission is called as "Edison effect". The filament must be heated to 2200 degree to emit useful no. of electrons. Because the electrons are negative charged and they repel each other, they bombard unacceptably large area of anode, and this is prevented by the cathode focusing cup which surrounds the filament. This focusing cup is made of nickel. Most of the X-ray tubes are now provided with two filaments; the larger filament is used for larger exposures. The filament should be never heated for long periods as it shortens the life of X-ray tube. Many X-ray circuits are supplied with automatic filament boosting circuit. When the X-ray circuit is made on but no exposure is being made, a "stand by" current heats the filament. This amount of filament heating is all required for fluoroscopy.

Tungsten vaporized from the filament gets deposited on the inner surface of glass wall of X-ray tube giving bronze colored "Sunburn".

LINE FOCUS PRINCIPLE (FIG. 1.3)

The focal spot is the area of tungsten anode that is bombarded by electrons from cathode. Most of the energy of electrons is converted into heat, with less than 1% being converted into X-rays. The heat is uniformly distributed over the focal spot; a large focal spot allows larger accumulation of heat leading to damage of target anode. For this reason, Line Focus Principle was introduced in 1918. The size and shape of electron streams are determined by dimensions of tungsten filament wire coil, the construction of focusing cup and position of filament in focusing cup. The electron stream bombards the target; the surface of Cup is inclined to form an angle. This is anode angle. It ranges from 6 to 20 degree. Thus as the angle of anode is made smaller, the apparent focal spot also becomes smaller.

THE ANODE

It is the positive electrode. It may be stationary or rotating. The tungsten is used as target material because of high atomic no. and high melting point. The small tungsten target must be bonded to much larger copper portion of the anode to facilitate heat dissipation and speed up its rate of cooling.

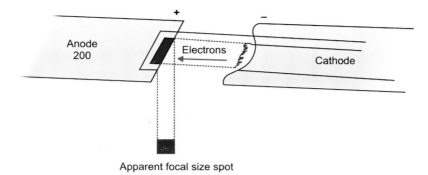

Apparent focal size spot

Fig. 1.3: The line focus principle

ROTATING ANODE

The ability of the X-ray tube to achieve high X-ray output is limited by the heat generated at the anode. The rotating anode principle is used to produce X-ray tubes capable of withstanding the heat generated by the large exposures. The rotating anode rotates at the speed of 3600 RPM. The purpose of rotating anode is to spread the heat produced during an exposure over a large area of anode. The heat generated in a solid tungsten disc is dissipated by radiating through the vacuum to the wall of tube, and then to surrounding oil and then the tube housing.

HEEL EFFECT

The intensity of X-ray beam that leaves the X-ray tube is not uniform throughout all the portions of the beam. The intensity of the beam depends on the angle at which the X-rays are emitted from the focal spot.

A. The intensity of film exposure on the anode side of X-ray tube is significantly less than that on the cathode side of tube, e.g. In X-ray of thoracic spine AP view the upper thoracic spine is focused under anode end where body is less thick. The cathode end of tube is over the lower thoracic spine where the thicker body structures will receive the increased exposure.

B. The heel effect is less noticeable when larger film focus distance is used.

C. For equal target film distances, the heel effect will be less for smaller films. This is concluded the intensity of the X-ray beam nearest the central ray is more uniform than that towards the periphery.

TUBE SHIELDING

The X-rays are scattered in all directions following collisions with various structures in and around the tube. The tube housing is lined with lead which absorbs primary and secondary X-rays. The effectiveness of full housing in limiting leakage radiation must meet the specifications listed in National Council on Radiation Protection. The leakage radiation measured at a distance of 1 meter from the source should not exceed 100 MR in an hour, when tube is operated at its maximum continuous rated current for the maximum rated tube potential. To prevent short circuiting between grounding wires and the tube, the space between them is filled with thick mineral oil. This oil has good electrical insulating and thermal cooling properties.

TUBE RATING CHARTS

It is necessary to speak of the total load that can be applied to an X-ray tube in terms of kilo voltage, milli amperes and exposure time. The load that can be safely accepted by X-ray tube is a function of heat energy produced during the exposure. The maximum temperature to which tungsten can be safely raised is generally considered to be 3000 degrees. The heat unit is defined as the product of current (MA) and KVP and time (sec) for single phase power supply. The term "Watt" is unit of power and it is the product of 1V times 1A.

$$1 W = 1V \times 1A$$

The term Kilowatt rating of an X-ray tube is commonly used to express the waiting of the tube to make single exposure of 0.1 sec. In considering tube rating, three characters are encountered.
1. The ability of the tube to withstand a single exposure.
2. The ability of the tube to function despite multiple rapid exposures.
3. The ability of the tube to withstand multiple exposures during several hours of heavy use.

The safe limit within which an X-ray tube can be operated for a single exposure can be easily determined by the tube rating chart supplied with all X-ray tubes.

METAL/CERAMIC X-RAY TABLES (FIG. 1.4)

Here instead of glass, metal or ceramic is used to insulate the high voltage parts of X-ray tube. Aluminum oxide is used as a ceramic insulator. The metal, when used in spite of glass for construction of X-ray tuber serves three purposes:
1. Less off focus radiation
2. Long tube life
3. Higher tube loading.

PROCESS OF X-RAY GENERATION

X-rays are produced by energy conversion when fast moving electrons interact with the tungsten anode. The X-rays are generated by two processes:

General Radiation/Bremsstrahlung

Here the high speed electrons lose energy in the target of X-ray tube.

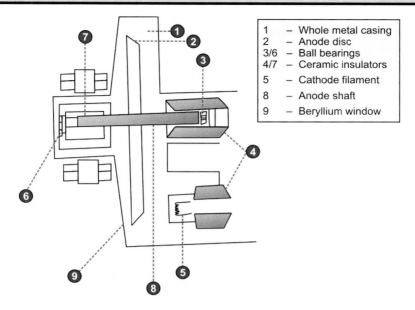

1	–	Whole metal casing
2	–	Anode disc
3/6	–	Ball bearings
4/7	–	Ceramic insulators
5	–	Cathode filament
8	–	Anode shaft
9	–	Beryllium window

Fig. 1.4: Model of super ceramic X-ray tube

Characteristic Radiation

It involves collision between high speed electrons and electrons in the shell of target. Tungsten atoms producing characteristic radiation.

X-RAY GENERATORS

It is the device that supplies electric power to the X-ray tube. The X-ray generator modifies the energy to meet the needs of X-ray tube. The tube requires electrical energy for two reasons:
1. To boil the electrons from the filament.
2. To accelerate these electrons from cathode to anode.

The mechanism of X-ray generator is usually continued in two separate compartments.
A. Control panel/console
B. Transformer assembly.

The control panel allows the operator to select the appropriate KVp, MA and exposure time for a particular X-ray. One exposure button (standby) readies the X-ray tube for exposure by heating the filament and rotating the anode and the other button starts the exposure. The timing mechanism terminates the exposure.

The second component is transformer assembly. It is a grounded metal box filled with oil. It contains a low voltage transformer for filament circuit and a high voltage transformer and a group of rectifier for the high voltage circuit.

The potential difference in these circuits may be as high as 150,000 V, so the transformers and rectifiers are immersed in oil. The oil serves as an insulator and prevents sparking between various components. Finally a transformer is a device that either increases or decreases the voltage in circuit. A rectifier changes alternating current into direct current.

A transformer consists of two wire coils wrapped around a closed core. The core is a simple rectangle with the wirings wound around opposite sides of rectangle (Fig. 1.5).

The circuit containing the first coil which is connected to the available electrical energy source is called as Primary circuit. The circuit containing the second coil from which comes the modified electric energy is called as Secondary circuit. When current flows through the primary coil, it creates a magnetic field within the core and this magnetic field induces a current in the secondary coil. Current only flows through the secondary circuit when magnetic field is changing, i.e. either increasing or decreasing.

For this reason, steady direct current in the primary coil cannot be used to produce a continuous current through the secondary coil.

Alternating current is used for a transformer because it is produced by a potential difference (voltage) that changes continuously in magnitude and periodically in polarity.

The most important characteristic of alternating current is that its voltage changes continuously, so it produces a continuously changing magnetic field. Therefore an alternating current in the primary cell of a transformer produces an alternating current as the secondary coil.

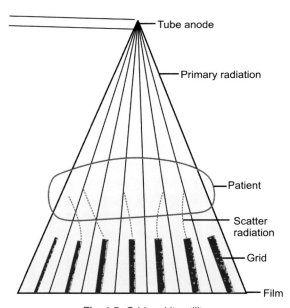

Fig. 1.5: Grid and its utility

LAWS OF TRANSFORMER

1. The voltage in two circuits is proportional to the no. of turns in the two coils.

$$\frac{Np}{Ns} = \frac{Vp}{Vs}$$

   Np= No. of turns in primary coil
   Ns= No. of turns in secondary coil
   Vp= Voltage in primary coil
   Vs= Voltage in secondary coil

2. The second law is simply a restatement of the law of conservation of energy. A transformer cannot create energy. An increase in voltage must be accompanied by a corresponding decrease in current. The product of voltage and current in the two circuits must be equal.

   Vp Ip= Vs Is
   Vp= Voltage in primary Cell
   Ip= Current in primary cell
   Vs= Voltage in secondary cell
   Is= Current in secondary cell
   The product of voltage and current is power.
   W = V x I Where W= Watt; I= Current in ampere; V= Volts

   A transformer with more turns in the secondary coil than primary coil increases voltage of the secondary circuit and it is a step up transformer. The other with few turns in secondary coil decreases the voltage and it is step down transformer. A transformer called as autotransformer supplies the supply voltage for both these circuits.

RECTIFICATION

It is the process of changing the alternating current into direct current. Device which produce this change is called Rectifier. When cathode is negative with respect to anode, electrons flow at high speed from cathode to anode and X-rays are produced. During the next half of the electrical cycle the anode is negative and the filament is positive, so electrons would flow away from target anode towards the cathode filament. This is not acceptable because such electrons would not produce X-rays and such electrons would heat the filament and reduce its life. By blocking the current flow in the inverse half of electrical cycle, the X-ray tube changes an alternating current into direct current. Because only half of the electrical wave is used to produce X-rays, this is half wave rectification.

RECTIFIER

A rectifier is a device that allows an electric current to flow in one direction but does not allow current to flow in other direction. Rectifiers are incorporated into X-ray circuit in series with the X-ray tube. High voltage rectifiers are of vacuum tube type or they can be of solid state composition. In 1965, high voltage silicon rectifiers were introduced and today most of X-ray generators use silicon rectifiers. The heart of solid state rectifier is a semiconductor, which is usually a piece of crystalline silicon. They are of two types the N type semiconductors and P type semiconductors.

Basic interaction between X-rays and matter: Only two interactions are important in diagnostic radiology, the photoelectric effect and Compton scattering. The photoelectric effect is the predominant interaction with low energy radiation and with high atomic no. absorber. It does not generate scatter radiation and reduces high contrast in the X-ray image but unfortunately exposes the patient great radiation. Compton scattering is responsible for almost all scatter radiation. The X-ray image contrast is less with computer reaction than with photoelectric effect.

ATTENUATION

It is the reduction in the intensity of X-ray beam as it traverses matter by enter the absorption of deflection of photons from the beam. The photons of X-ray beam enter a patient with a uniform distribution and emerge out in a specific pattern of distribution. The transmitted and attenuated photons are equally important. If all the photons are transmitted the film will be black and if all the photons were attenuated the film would be uniformly white. The image formation depends on differential attenuation between the tissues. Some tissues attenuate more X-ray than other tissues and the size of this differential determine the X-ray image. In human body, the X-ray attenuation is greater in bone than other parts.

SCATTER RADIATION

It detracts the film quality and contributes no useful information. There are three factors determining the quantity of scatter radiation.
1. Kvp
2. Body Part thickness
3. Field size

The scatter radiation is maximum with high Kvp techniques, large field and thick body parts. We don't have control over body part thickness and field size. The only variable we can control is Kvp.

FILTERS

Filtering is the process of shaping the X-ray beam to increase the ratio of photons useful for imaging to those photons that decrease image contrast. Filters are usually sheets of metal which reduces the patient's radiation dose. In a radiological examination the X-ray beam is filtered by absorber at three different levels:

1. The X-ray tube and its housing (inherent filtration)
2. Sheets of metal placed in the path of beam (added filtration)
3. The patient.

Aluminum is usually placed as the filter material for diagnostic radiology. Most high energy photons are transmitted through aluminum while low energy photons are absorbed by photoelectric interactions. National council on radiation for protection and measurement has recommended an equivalent of 2.5 mm of aluminum permanent filtration for diagnostic X-ray.

COLLIMATORS

There are three types of X-ray beam restrictors- aperture diaphragms; cones and collimators. Their basic function is to regulate the size and shape of X-ray beam. Closely collimated beams have two advantages- first a smaller area of patient is exposed and because area is a square function, a decrease of one half in X-ray beam diameter affects a fourfold decrease in patient exposure. Second well collimated beams generate less radiation and thus improve film quality.

GRIDS

It consists of a series of lead foil strips separated by X-ray transparent spaces. It was invented by Dr Gustave Bucky in 1913 and it is still most effective way of removing scatter radiation from large radiographic field. Primary radiation is oriented in the same axis as the lead strips and passes between them to reach the film unaffected by the grid. Scatter radiation arises from many points within the patient and it is multidirectional so most of it is absorbed by the lead strips and only a small amount passes between. Grid ratio is defined as the ratio between the height of the lead strips and the distance between them. Grids are mainly used to improve contrast by absorbing secondary radiation/scatter radiation before it reaches the film.

The primary disadvantage of grids is that they increase the amount of radiation that the patient receives. Another disadvantage is that they require careful centering of the X-ray tube because of the danger of grid cut off. Grid cut off is the loss of primary radiation occurs when the images of lead strips are projected wider then double width.

MOUNTING GRIDS

It was invented by Dr Hollis E Potter in 1920 and it was called as Potter Bucky grid. Grids are moved to blur out the shadows cast by the lead strips. Three grids move continuously back and forth or 1 to 3 cm throughout the exposure. These grids eliminate grid lines from the film. The disadvantages of moving grids are:
1. They are expensive
2. Subject to failure
3. Vibrates the X-ray tube

4. Puts a limit on the minimum exposure time so they move slowly
5. It increases patient's radiation dose.

The other way of reducing the scatter radiation without increasing the patient radiation is air gap technique. The closer the patient is to film, the greater is the concentration of scatter per unit area. With air gap the concentration decreases therefore more scattered photons miss the film.

FLUOROSCOPIC IMAGING

X-rays were discovered because of their ability to cause fluorescence and first X-ray image observed fluoroscopically. Initial fluoroscope consisted of X-ray tube, X-ray table and fluoroscopic screen. The fluorescent material was copper automated zinc cadmium sulfide that emitted the light on yellow green spectrum. A sheet of lead glass covered the screen so the radiologist could stare directly into the screen without having the X-ray beam striking his eyes. Screen fluoroscopy was so faint that the examination was carried out in dark room by radiologist who had dark adopted his eyes by wearing goggles, for 10 to 30 minutes prior to examination. The solution came to above problem in the form of X-ray image intensifier developed in 1950s.

The Design of Image Intensifier

The X-ray tube is a vacuum tube which contains:
1. Input phosphor and photocathode
2. Electrostatic focusing lens
3. Accelerating anode
4. Output phosphor.

After an X-ray beam passes through the patient, it enters the image intensifier tube. The input fluorescent screen absorbs X-ray photons and converts their energy into light photons. The light photons strike the photocathode, causing it to emit photoelectrons. These electrons are immediately draws away from photocathode by high potential difference between it and the accelerating anode. As the electrons flow from the cathode towards the anode they are focused by an electrostatic lens which guides them to the output fluorescent screen without distracting their geometric configuration.

The electrons strike the output screen which emits the light photons that carry the fluoroscopic image to the eye of the observer. Thus in the intensifier tube, the image is carried first by X-ray photons, then by light photons next by electrons and finally by light photons. The input fluorescent screen in image intensifies due to cesium iodide which is deposited in a thin aluminum substrate by a process called vapor deposition. The image quality is better with cesium iodide input screen that's why of vertical orientation of crystals, a greater packing density and a more favorable atomic number. The thickness of phosphor layer is 0.1 mm. The principal advantage of thinner phosphor layer combined with needle shaped crystals is improved resolution. The resolution of cesium iodide image intensifier will be about four lines per mm.

The photocathode is photosensitive metal commonly combination of antimony and cesium compounds. When light from the flavescent screen strikes the photocathode, photoelectrons are emitted in number proportional to the brightness of the screen. The photocathode is directly applied to the cesium iodide input phosphor.

ELECTROSTATIC FOCUSING LENS

The lens is made up of a series of positively charged electrodes that are usually plated on the inside surface of the glass envelope. These electrodes focus the electron beam from photocathode toward the output phosphor. Electron focusing inverts and reverses the image. This is called point inversion that's why all the electrons pass through a common focal point on their way to the output phosphor.

ACCELERATING ANODE

It is located in the neck of image intensifier tube. Its function is to accelerate the electrons emitted from photocathode toward the output screen. The anode has a positive potential of 25 to 35 Kv relative to the photocathode, so it accelerates electrons to a tremendous velocity.

OUTPUT PHOSPHOR

It is silver activated zinc cadmium sulfide. The crystal size and layer thickness are reduced to maintain resolution in magnified image. A thin layer of aluminum is plated on to the fluorescent screen to prevent light from moving retrograde through the tube and activating the photocathode. The glass tube of IIT is about 2 to 4 mm thick enclosed in a lead lived container. The output phosphor image is viewed either directly through a series of lenses and mirror or indirectly through closed circuit television. Large field of view image intensifier tubes- the development of digital angiography was associated with a need for large image intensifier tubes that could image a large area of patient. Those image intensifier tubes with diameter of 12, 14 and 16 inches are now available to meet this need. The magnification factor with the small field can be helpful when fluoroscopy is used to guide delicate invasive procedures such as percutaneous biliary and nephrostomy.

CLOSED CIRCUIT TELEVISION

Here the signals are transferred from one component to the next through cables and not through the air. A lens system or a fiber optic system conveys the fluoroscopic image from the output phosphor of the image intensifier to the video camera, where it is converted into a series of electrical pulses called the video signal. This signal is transmitted through a cable to the camera control unit, where it is amplified and then forwarded through another cable to the TV monitor. The monitor converts the video signal back into the original image for direct viewing.

The TV image is made up of thousand tiny dots of different brightness each contributing a minute bit to the total picture.

RADIATION PROTECTION

In 1928, the second international congress of radiology appointed a committee to define the Roentgen as a unit of exposure. The harmful effects of radiation fall in two categories:
1. Somatic- Harmful to the person being irradiated.
2. Genetic- Those harmful to future generations.

In actual practice radiation level should be kept at the lowest practicable level and one should not think of permissible doses as being perfectly safe. The most important somatic effect of radiation is carcinogenesis and leukoderma. The genetic effects of radiation are more frightening than somatic ones because they may manifest themselves for several generations.

RADIATION UNITS

There are three units the Roentgen, the Rad and the Rem.

The roentgen is defined as a unit of radiation exposure that will liberate a charge of $2.5 \times 10 - 4$ coulombs per kilo = gram of air.

The rad is the unit of absorbed dose. One rad is equal to the radiation necessary to deposit energy of 100 ergs in 1 gram of irradiated material (100 erg/gm).

The Gray (Gy) is the SI unit of absorbed dose. One Gray is defined as to be radiation necessary to deposit energy of one joule in 1 kg of tissue. One Gray is equivalent to 100 rads.

The rem is a unit absorbed dose equivalent. The rem is a unit used only as radiation protection. Its SI unit is Sievert.

All individuals exposed to radiation in low doses. In an attempt to make some comparison in the risk assessment for all types of exposure, the concept of effective dose equivalent (H_E) has been developed.

Medical Radiation

The concept of effective dose equivalent is particularly useful while describing medical X-ray exposures. There are two categories of medical radiation: diagnostic medical X-rays and nuclear medicine. The estimated annual effective dose equivalent from diagnostic X-ray examination is 0.39 MSV.

DOSE LIMITING RECOMMENDATIONS

There are four classes of individuals:
1. Occupationally exposed individuals
2. The general public

3. Trainees under 18 years of age
4. Embryo fetus.

Occupational Exposure

It is knowledgeable group, who knows risk involved and their no. are relatively small. So his exposure does not contribute appreciably to genetically significant dose. The maximum permissible does is larger for this group than other people. The stochastic effect of radiation exposure is defined as air effect in which the probability of occurrence increases with increasing absorbed dose, but the severity of effect does not depend on the magnitude to the absorbed dose, e.g. Cancers and genetic effects.

A no stochastic effect of radiation exposure is defined as a somatic effect that increases in severity with increasing absorbed dose. These are degenerative effects severe enough to be clinically significant such as organ atrophy and fibrosis, e.g. Lens opacification, blood changes and increased sperm production.

For occupational exposures, the NCRP recommends an annual effective dose equivalent limit of 5 rem (50 MSV). For avoidance of non stochastic effects recommended annual dose equivalent limits are 15 rem (150 MSV) for the lens of eye and 50 rem (500 MSV) for other organs.

An individual lifetime effective dose equivalent in rems should not exceed the value of his/her age in years.

Public (Non-occupational) Exposure

They have no knowledge of the risk involved, receives no compensation for taking a risk. When a member of general population enters a radiating area, he becomes an occasionally exposed individual. Large number of individuals could be involved which would have a greater impact on the genetically significant dose. For all these reasons, the dose limit for the occasionally exposed is 0.5 rem/year or 1/10 if maximal permissible dose for the occupationally exposed.

Trainees Under 18 years of Age

The NCRP recommends that exposure to these trainees should result in an annual effective dose equivalent of less than 0.1 rem.

Embryo Fetus Exposure

The NCRP recommends a total dose of 0.5 rem (50 MSV) for th embryo fetus. Once pregnancy becomes known exposure of embryo fetus should be no greater than 0.05 rem (0.5 MSV) in any month.

PROTECTIVE BARRIERS

The distance, time and barriers are used to control radiation exposure levels.

Distance is obviously an effective method that's why beams intensity is governed by inverse general law. Exposures can be controlled with time in various ways.

Barriers are designated as either primary or secondary depending on whether they protect from primary radiation of stray radiation.

The exposure from primary beams can be calculated by multyplying the workload, use factor, occupancy factor and inverse square of the distance by an R output at 1 m for each MA of workload. If this exposure exceeds permissible levels, then a barrier is required. Barrier thickness is calculated in two ways:

1. With precalculated tables
2. With half value layer of lead or concrete.

The half value layer (HVL) is the thickness of a specific substances that when introduced into the path of a beam of radiation, reduces the exposure by one half.

A secondary barrier is required only when the useful beam cannot be directed at particular wall. Secondary barrier protect against scatter and leakage radiation. For scatter radiation the exposure is assumed to the attenuated by a factor of 1000 (i.e. reduced to 0.001 at a distance 1 ms each for each right angle scattering).

RECOMMENDED FOR FURTHER READING

1. David Sutton- Textbook of Radiology

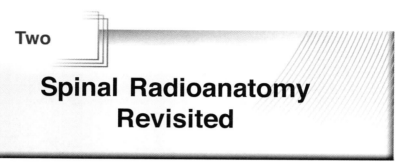

Two

Spinal Radioanatomy Revisited

Sachin Pathak, Pradeep Krishnan, Vishal Piparia, Bhavin Jhankaria

INTRODUCTION

- Selective nerve block for pain management requires injection of a local anesthetic into a desired nerve/branch of nerve under image guidance [fluoroscopy/ultrasound/CT scan].
- Fluoroscopy is commonly used in spinal nerve blocks and for cervical/thoracic/lumbar discographies. Fluoroscopy guided nerve block is performed as a diagnostic as well as a prognostic procedure.
- This involves guiding the needle under fluoroscopic guidance towards a target point specific for the type of block.
- For this, knowledge of spinal radio anatomy and orientation of AP/lateral and oblique views of the spine is essential.
- The vertebral column is composed of a series of 31 vertebrae. There are 7 cervical, 12 thoracic, and 5 lumbar vertebrae. The sacrum is composed of 5 fused vertebrae, and 2 coccygeal vertebrae which are sometimes fused.
- In the normal adult there are four curvatures in the vertebral column in an anteroposterior plane. These serve to align the head with a vertical line through the pelvis. In the thoracic and sacral regions, these curves are oriented concave anteriorly and each is known as a kyphosis.
- In the lumbar and cervical regions the curves are convex anteriorly and each is known as a lordosis.
- A curvature of the vertebral column in the mediolateral plane can occur pathologically and is known as a scoliosis.

STRUCTURE OF A TYPICAL VERTEBRA (FIGS 2.1 TO 2.4)

- Each vertebra is composed of a body anteriorly and a neural arch posteriorly. The arch encloses an opening, the vertebral foramen, which helps to form a canal in which the spinal cord is housed.
- Protruding from the posterior extreme of each neural arch is a spinous process and extending from the lateral edges of each arch are transverse processes.

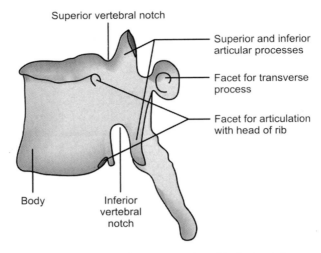

Fig. 2.1: Diagrammatic representation of typical vertebrae

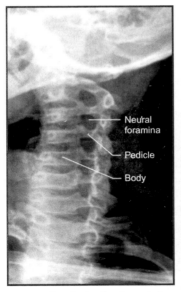

Fig. 2.2: Cervical spine-lateral view-showing neural foramina and pedicle

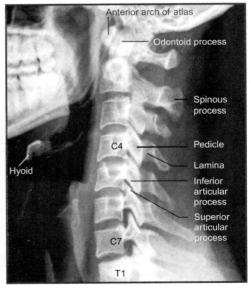

Fig. 2.3: Cervical spine-lateral view-parts of vertebrae

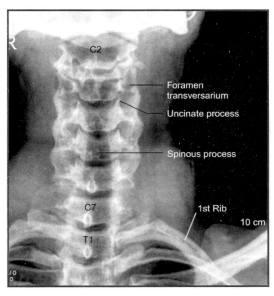

Fig. 2.4: Cervical spine-AP view-parts of vertebrae

- The neural arch of each vertebra is divided into component parts by these processes. The parts of the neural arch between the spinous and transverse processes are known as the lamina and the parts of the arch between the transverse processes and the body are the pedicles.
- At the point where the lamina and pedicles meet, each vertebra contains two superior articular facets and two inferior articular facets. The former pair of facets form articulations, which are synovial joints, with the two inferior articular facets of the vertebra immediately above (or the skull, in the case of the first cervical vertebra).
- The pedicle of each vertebra is notched at its superior and inferior edges. Together the notches from two contiguous vertebras form an opening, the intervertebral foramen, through which spinal nerves pass.

The first and second cervical vertebrae are atypical. The first cervical vertebra is known as the atlas, and it is remarkable for having no body. It contains an anterior tubercle instead. Its superior articular facets articulate with the occipital condyles of the skull and are oriented in a roughly parasagittal plane. The head thus moves forward and backwards on this vertebra.

- The second cervical vertebra contains a prominent odontoid process, or dens, which projects superiorly from its body. It articulates with the anterior tubercle of the atlas, forming a pivotal joint. Side to side movements of the head take place about this joint.
- The seventh cervical vertebra is sometimes considered atypical since it lacks a bifid spinous process.

Thoracic Vertebrae (Figs 2.5 and 2.6)

- The unique characteristic of thoracic vertebrae is articular facets for the ribs. Each vertebra contains two pairs of these costal demifacets on its body and one on each transverse process. Typical ribs articulate with the inferior demifacet and transverse process of a thoracic vertebra and the superior demifacet of the vertebra below it.
- The 11th and 12th thoracic vertebrae are sometimes considered atypical because they lack a superior costal demifacet. The 11th and 12th ribs thus articulate only with the 11th and 12th thoracic vertebrae, respectively.

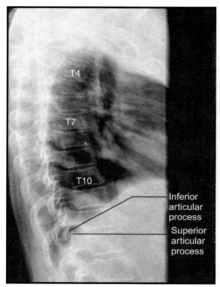

Fig. 2.5: Thoracic spine-lateral view-showing articular process

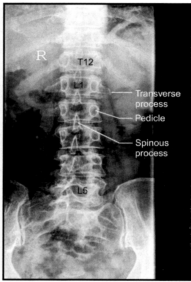

Fig. 2.6: Thoracic lumbar spine-AP view-various parts

Lumbar Vertebrae (Figs 2.1 and 2.6)

Lumbar vertebrae are characterized by massive bodies and robust spinous and transverse processes.

- Their articular facets are oriented somewhat parasagittally, which is thought to contribute to the large range of anteroposterior bending possible between lumbar vertebrae (Fig. 2.7).

SCOTTY DOG (FIGS 2.8 AND 2.9)

Oblique Radiograph of the Lumbar Spine "The Scotty Dog" Appearance

On oblique radiographs, the posterior elements form the appearance of a "Scotty dog", where the superior articular process resemble the ear, the pedicle

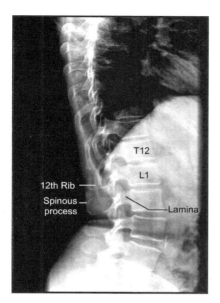

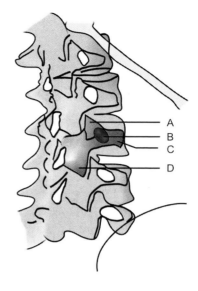

Fig. 2.7: X-ray thoracolumbar spine-lateral view showing parts of vertebrae

Fig. 2.8: Diagrammatic representation-scotty dog: A-Sup. art. process (ear of dog); B-Eye of dog-pedicle; C-Transverse process-(Nose of dog); D-Inf. art. process-(Lower leg of dog)

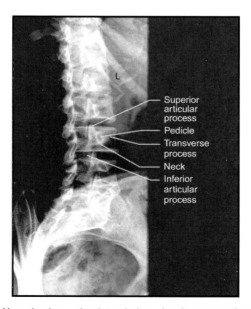

Fig. 2.9: X-ray-lumbar spine-lateral view-showing parts of scotty dog: Sup. art. process, transverse process; Inf. art. process

forms the eye, the transverse process forms the nose and the inferior articular process forms the lower leg of the dog. The pars interarticularis forms the neck of the dog.

Sacrum (Fig. 2.10)

- The sacrum consists of five fused vertebrae. It articulates with the fifth lumbar vertebra above and the coccyx below, and with the iliac bones on either side.
- In addition to its characteristic shape, it contains both anterior and posterior foramina through which the anterior and posterior rami of the spinal nerves pass.

Intervertebral Joints

- Adjacent vertebrae are connected by three types of intervertebral articulations. Synovial joints are formed between the inferior articular facets of one vertebrae and the superior articular facets of the vertebrae below.
- These joints are extensively re-enforced by different ligaments.
- These ligaments connect the tips of the spinous processes (supraspinous ligaments), the base of the spinous processes (interspinous ligaments), and the transverse processes (intertransversalis ligaments).
- In addition the laminas of adjacent vertebrae are bound together by a ligamentum flavum.

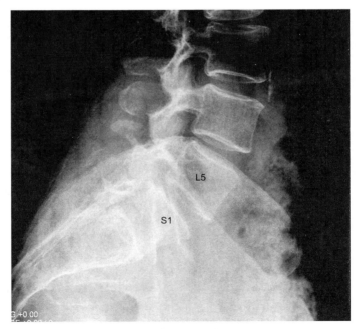

Fig. 2.10: Sacrum and coccyx

- The bodies of adjacent vertebrae are connected by specialized cartilaginous joints known as intervertebral discs. Each disc is composed of a central core of gelatinous material, known as the nucleus pulposus, and a surrounding series of fibrous rings known as the annulus fibrosis. In most individuals, the fibers of the annulus fibrosus effectively resist this load, but in some people they do not and the nucleus pulposus is forced out of the disc, or is herniated.
- A herniated nucleus pulposus can have a profound effect on the adjacent spinal nerves.
- Two ligaments connect the vertebral bodies anteriorly and posteriorly and thereby re-enforce the intervertebral disc. The anterior longitudinal ligament is strong and robust throughout but the posterior longitudinal ligament becomes thin and narrow in the lumbar region.
- This change in structure of the posterior longitudinal ligament is part of the reason that the overwhelming majority of disc herniations occur posteriorly in the lumbar region.

The Spinal Cord

- The spinal cord proper begins at the level of the foramen magnum of the skull and ends at the level of the L1/L2 intervertebral joint. There it tapers to a cone-shaped ending known as the conus medullaris. A stalk of pia mater, the filum terminale attaches it to the end of the dura mater at S2. All of the roots of the spinal nerves from L2 to the lowest coccygeal nerve pass caudal to the conus medullaris to exit at their respective intervertebral foramina. This mass of spinal roots within the spinal canal (in the subarachnoid space) is known as the cauda equina. Thus, the area of the subarachnoid space below the L2 vertebra (typically L4) is considered a safe place to insert a needle to sample cerebrospinal fluid, since only nerve roots and not spinal cord are found there.
- Likewise, the posterior protrusion of a herniated lower lumbar intervertebral disc, while not pressing on the spinal cord, can compress a lumbar nerve root, causing severe pain or physical dysfunction in distinct areas of the lower limb.

The Intervertebral Canal

- It is situated between adjacent pedicles which form its upper and lower boundaries. The intervertebral canal is widest superiorly, narrowing inferiorly. The intervertebral canal narrows with extension as the facets slide over each other.
- The cervical intervertebral canal is oriented anterolaterally at 45 degrees to the sagittal plane and is best demonstrated using the oblique radiographic projection.
- Lateral radiographs are appropriate for demonstrating the cervical neural foramina (Fig. 2.11).

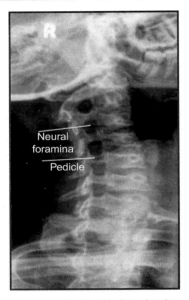

Fig. 2.11: X-ray cervical spine-lateral view-showing neural foramina

- The dorsal root ganglia, epidural fat, the spinal nerves and the blood vessels are found in the intervertebral canal.
- In the thoracic and lumbar regions the neural elements traverse the superior part of the intervertebral canal. The superior part of the cervical neural canal contains foraminal veins, while the nerve root ganglia lie in the inferior part.

RECOMMENDED FOR FURTHER READING

1. David Sutton- Textbook of Radiology

Three

Neurolytic Agents and Neurodestructive Techniques

RP Gehdoo

INTRODUCTION

Injection of neurolytic agents to destroy nerves and interrupt pain pathways as well as neurodestructive techniques have been extensively used to achieve 'permanent' analgesia in the cases of advanced chronic pain patients by the pain practitioners since the early part of the 20th Century. The results of such injections are essentially the same as nerve sectioning, although the effect is usually seen for only 3 to 6 months. Schloesser, in 1903[1], used alcohol for the first time in the cases of trigeminal neuralgia. A neurolytic sympathetic block was used for providing the anginal and abdominal pain relief by Swetlow[2] in 1926. Intrathecal alcohol neurolysis for the intractable pain relief was used for the first time by Digliotti[3] in 1933. However, the use of neurolysis has decreased significantly in recent years due to advances in spinal analgesia and increased life expectancies in patients with cancer. In 1851, Arnott[4] reported the application of cold in relieving cancer pain. Smith and Fay[5] in 1939 reported finding regression of tumor following localized freezing. But still, neurolysis continues to be an attractive option for pain control in many cancer patients. Neurolysis is indicated inpatients with severe, intractable pain in whom less aggressive maneuvers are ineffective or intolerable because of either poor physical condition or the development of side effects.

Various chemical agents used for the purpose of neurolysis are alcohol, phenol, glycerol, chlorocresol, ammonium salts and hypertonic saline. For the neurodestruction techniques, cryoablation and of late, radiofrequency lesioning has been used in the pain practice.

MECHANISM OF ACTION

As soon as the neurolytic agents like alcohol or phenol come in contact with the nerve fiber, there is an increase in the endoneurial fluid pressure secondary to the mast cell degranulation and release of vasoactive substances. This elevated pressure causes stretching of the perineurium and compression of perineurial vessels. This leads to ischemia of nerve fiber and interruption of nerve impulses. Adequate amount of wallerian degeneration should be accompanied to get good results.

Types of Neurolytic Agents and Neurodestructive Techniques are as follows

A. Chemical Neurolytic Agents: Alcohol, Phenol, Glycerol, Ammonium salts, and Hypertonic saline
B. Cryoablation
C. Radiofrequency Lesioning

Chemical Neurolytic Agents

The neurolytic agents commonly used for chemical neurolysis include Ethyl alcohol, phenol, chlorocresol, ammonium salts and hypertonic saline etc.

1. *Ethyl alcohol:* It is a clear, colorless solution. It absorbs water on exposure to air. It is stable at room temperature and hypobaric to CSF. It spreads quite rapidly from the injection site and requires 12 to 24 hours before the effects of the injection can be assessed. Ninety to ninety-eight percent of the injected alcohol is rapidly metabolized by oxidation in the liver principally by the enzyme alcohol dehydrogenase.

   This is available in various concentrations from 50 to 97%. The minimum concentration required for neurolysis has not been established. However, Labat G[6] reported in 1933 that an injection of 33.3% alcohol produced satisfactory analgesia in the treatment of painful disorders.

   Its mechanism of nerve destruction is similar to phenol. It extracts cholesterol, phospholipids and cerebrosides from the nervous tissue and causes precipitations of lipoproteins and mucoproteins.[7] This initiates Wallerian degeneration and neurolysis. Whenever intrathecal alcohol is given, similar changes are noted in the nerve rootlets. There can be a minimal focal inflammation of meninges and patchy areas of demyelination in the dorsal column, Lissauer's tract and dorsal root.[8] When sympathetic chain comes in contact with alcohol, the ganglion cells get destroyed.[9-11] This blocks all postganglionic fibers to all effector organs. Following its injection, the patient complains of severe burning pain along the nerve's distribution which may last for a minute and is subsequently replaced by a warm, numb sensation. To overcome this pain, an injection of local anesthetic agent prior and following the alcohol injection should be done.

   It is used for neurolysis at cranial nerves, intrathecal injection, sympathetic chain and chemical hypophysectomy.

   Usually it is given at a dose of 20 to 25 ml of 50% alcohol on either side in case of advanced upper GI malignancy cases, while in the varying doses of 0.25 to 2 ml of absolute (97%) alcohol in all other cranial and sympathetic nerves or ganglions.

2. *Phenol:* Phenol is a chemical composite containing carbolic acid, phenic acid, phenylic acid, phenyl hydroxide, hydroxybenzene, and oxyben-

zene. In its pure state, it is colorless and poorly soluble. Shelf life exceeds one year when the solution is refrigerated and not exposed to light. Phenol turns red on exposure to sunlight and air because of oxidation. A reddish tinge. It is available as a sterile solution and can be prepared as a 6.7% solution in water.

Usually it is available in concentrations ranging from 4 to 10%. Since phenol is hyperbaric, it will settle if injected into a liquid medium such as the cerebrospinal fluid-containing subarachnoid space. It is highly soluble in organic solvents such as alcohol and glycerine. The addition of small amounts of glycerol or water soluble radiopaque contrast material may increase the concentration to 15%. The solution can be diluted with saline and is compatible when mixed with radio-contrast dyes. The glycerine mixed phenol is thick solution and needs to be injected through a needle not less than 20 Gz. When mixed with glycerine, it slowly diffuses from the solution. This property of phenol can be taken into advantages, when injected intrathecally because it allows for limited spread and is localized in the area that needed to be destroyed. When mixed with water, it has a wider spread, causing a bigger area of nerve destruction. Aqueous solution of phenol is more potent than the glycerine solution. The choice of diluents depends upon the extent of neurolysis desired. The use of higher concentrations of phenol might predispose to a higher incidence of vascular injury. It is metabolized in the liver by conjugation to glucuronides and oxidation to equinol compounds or to carbon dioxide and water. Excretion of metabolites is via the kidneys.

Phenol causes non-selective neurolysis by denaturing proteins of axons and perineural blood vessels.[12] There is loss of cellular fatty elements, separation of the myelin sheath from the axon, and axonal edema.[13] The degeneration after contact with solution takes about 14 days and regeneration is completed in about 14 weeks. However, phenol is not as effective as alcohol at destroying the nerve cell body and its blocking effect tends to be less profound and of shorter duration than alcohol. At a concentration of 2 to 3% in saline, phenol seems to spare motor function. The efficacy of 3% phenol in saline is comparable to that of 40% alcohol. It acts as a local anesthetic in lower concentrations and as a neurolytic in higher concentrations. The effects of the block cannot be evaluated until after 24 to 48 hours, to allow time for the local anesthetic effect to dissipate. The neurolytic effect may be clinically evident only after 3 to 7 days. If inadequate pain relief is obtained after two weeks, this may indicate incomplete neurolysis and requires repetition of the procedure. The subsequent fibrosis that occurs following phenol injection makes nerve regeneration more difficult, but not impossible. Nerve regeneration can occur as long as the nerve cell body is intact, at a rate of 1 to 3 mm per day. Nerve arborization and neuroma formation can occur at the site of nerve disruption and can be a focus of a neuropathic type of pain. Phenol can be injected intrathecally and epidurally. Phenol in glycerine is hyperbaric compared to the CSF. It can be used also for paravertebral somatic block, peripheral nerve blocks, in epidural, peripheral nerve roots, intrathecal and cranial nerves and sympathetic blocks.

Phenol has systemic side effects including central nervous system stimulation, cardiovascular depression, nausea, and vomiting. Systemic doses of more than 5 grams can cause convulsive seizures and central nervous system depression. Doses less than 100 mg are less likely to cause serious side effects.

3. *Glycerol:* It is a mild neurolytic agent used preferably for the Gasserian ganglion block, as it was found to preserve the facial sensations in most of the cases. It is usually used as 100% solution in 0.5 to 2 ml dose. Due to a poor control of spread in the area close to the subarachnoid space, it is not used in the intrathecal injection.

The mechanism of it's action is not completely understood. However, it appears to affect primarily damaged myelinated axons. Injection in the vicinity of the nerve causes perineural damage, while intra-neural injection results in Schwann cell edema, axonolysis, and Wallerian degenarion. Intra-neural injection destroys all the fibers.

4. *Ammonium salts:* Ammonium salts used for long-term pain relief. It is usually available at a concentration of 10%. At this concentration, a neuronal degeneration, including C-fibers neurolysis, appears with a success of 40%. Interestingly, it has been found that a 10% solution provides adequate analgesia without a significant motor block.

These salts produce an acute degenerative neuropathy with obliteration of C-fibers and with a very small effect on A-fibers. However, the degeneration is nonselective and may affect all types of fibers.

Complications due to ammonium salts injection are transient and include nausea and headache. Paresthesia and burning sensation may occur in 30% of patients at doses 500 mgs of ammonium salts, lasting 2 to 14 days.

5. *Hypertonic saline or normal saline:* The use of hypertonic saline by intrathecal injection to treat intractable pain was first reported by Hitchcock[14] in 1967. The most commonly used solution is the 10% aqueous solution and it is readily available. It is usually given intrathecally as 40 to 60 ml of normal saline injection, after withdrawing an equal amount of CSF (a very distressing procedure).

Its mechanism of neurolysis is not well elaborated. Normal saline usually is thought to act specifically on C-fibers, sparing larger fibers of sensory, motor, and autonomic functions. Cold hypertonic saline produces C-fiber neurolysis with a success of 30%. It causes severe pain on injection and local anesthetic is first injected before the saline solution. When injected intrathecally, it seems to produce it's action by an intrathecal shift of water with extracellular change in osmolarity. Intrathecal injection of hypertonic saline can cause an increase in the intracranial pressure, increase in blood pressure, heart rate and respiratory rate.

Duration of the pain relief is normally short-lived, may be from 10 to 25 days. Rarely, one may find a relief extending to a couple of months.

Cardiac complications have been seen during and after saline injection. Complications consists of tachycardia, premature ventricular contractions and myocardial infarction, localized paresis (which may last for many hours), paresthesia (which may last for many weeks), hemiplegia, pulmonary edema, pain in the ear, vestibular disturbances, and loss of sphincter control with sacral anesthesia.

Indications for Chemical Neurolysis

1. Management of chronic, intractable, non-terminal pain that are not responsive to other modalities.
2. Treatment of cancer pain in those patients who have short life expectancy (less than a year).
3. Alternative management to treat spasticity in order to improve balance, gait, self-care, and global rehabilitation. An important difference between neurolytic blocks for pain relief versus spasticity is that motor or mixed nerves are targeted preferentially in the management of spastic disorders.

Complications of Chemical Neurolysis

i. *Skin and other tissues:* There is a necrosis and sloughing of the skin and other non-target tissues, mainly due to damage of the vascular supply, and subsequent chronic trauma to denervated tissue. Necrosis of muscles, blood vessels, and other soft tissues has also been reported.

ii. *Neuritis:* The incidence of neuritis is up to 10%. It is caused by partial destruction of somatic nerve and subsequent regeneration. It is clinically manifested as hyperesthesia and dysesthesia that may be worse than the original pain problem. It is one of the limiting factors in the use of chemical neurolysis.

iii. *Anesthesia dolorosa:* This is a poorly understood condition whereby the patient complains of distressing numbness caused by an imbalance in afferent input. It is caused by long-term loss of afferent input and the resultant CNS changes. Management of this problem is pharmacotherapy with the use of tricyclic antidepressants, major antipsychotic tranquilizers, and anticonvulsants.

iv. *Prolonged motor paralysis:* This can be a major complication, that occurs infrequently and is usually temporary.

v. *Perineal and sexual dysfunction:* This is another fearsome complication that can occur temporarily. About 1.4% and 0.2% of patients will have bowel or bladder dysfunction at one week and one month, respectively.

vi. *Systemic complications:* These include hypotension secondary to sympathetic block and systemic toxic reactions, heart rate and rhythm disturbances, blood pressure changes, and CNS excitation and depression.

Cryoablation

Pain relief from the destruction of nerves following exposure to extreme cold is called cryoanalgesia. Smith and Fay[15] in 1939 reported a tumor regression following localized freezing. Lloyd and coworkers[16] in 1976 used this method for pain relief and coined the term "cryoanalgesia".

The major advantage of this procedure is the absence of neuritis or neuroma formation, and prolonged analgesia with reversible effect unlike chemical neurolysis[17] and to a certain extent, radiofrequency lesioning.[18,19] It has no systemic side effects and produces minimal tissue damage. It can be performed as an outpatient procedure. The pain relief might last from 2 weeks to 5 months.

Cryoablation involves inducing profound hypothermia over nerve fiber (at the contact point). A prolongation of action potentia is seen, when nerve is cooled to 5° C. Unmyelinated fibers require a lower temperature. Cryolesioning is done by freezing of a small nerve segment with a 2 mm probe cooled at – 60° C by rapid expansion of pressurized nitrous oxide from its tip. The probe is left in contact with the nervous tissue for 60 to 90 seconds and then allowed to thaw for another 45 to 60 seconds before being removed. An ice ball 2 to 4 mm in diameter is formed that freezes the nerve and completely damages the nerve fiber. Endoneurial fluid pressure is elevated up to 20 mm Hg within 90 minutes. It reduces over next 24 hours and then increases again, to reach a plateau after 6 days secondary to changes of wallerian degeneration.

It is particularly useful in the management of chronic pain syndrome, when other modalities of pain relief are unacceptable to patients such as surgery or device implantation, too difficult to perform, have a high incidence of complications or side effects, or has been ineffective. The techniques has been utilized in the treatment of various types of neuralgias (fascial, intercostal, post-therapeutic, post-traumatic), myofascial trigger point pain, post-surgical pain, cancer pain, neuroma, phantom limb pain, cervicogenic headache, cervicalgia, thoracic, lumbar and coccygeal pain. These can be usually done as an outpatient procedure, readily acceptable to patients, minimal complications, and an effective alternative to pharmacologic pain killers.

The therapeutic effectiveness of cryoablation is difficult to predict. There is wide patient to patient variability depending upon the site of lesioning, nature of the pain problem, psychologic make up of the individual, and experience of the operator. Across the board, the effectiveness may vary from 3 to 1000 days.

It has a special N_2O delivery system that allows safe delivery of the gas up to 850 psi to the gas expansion orifice in the tip of the cryoprobe (14, 16, 18 gauge). Generally, the gas is delivered at an operating pressure of 600 psi. The minimum temperature at the tip of the probe can rapidly reach to – 60° C.

The commonly encountered complications are Frostbite and depigmentation of skin, sensory and motor damage and damage to the adjacent structures due to movements or mal-positioning of the probe.

Radiofrequency Lesioning

Radiofrequency lesioning is the application of electrical current to promote the thermocoagulation, leading ultimately to the nerve destruction. It is used to ablate pain pathways in the trigeminal ganglion, spinal cord, dorsal root entry zone, dorsal root ganglion, sympathetic chain, facet joints, failed back pain syndrome and peripheral nerves.[20-24] Since it causes nerve destruction, this technique is utilized only as end of the line therapeutic modality when other measures have failed. Fluoroscopic guidance is a requirement for proper needle placement. The patient should also be informed of the risks and benefits of the procedure and a written informed consent must be signed in front of a witness.

The mechanism of action of RF lesioning is as follows: Frictional heat is generated by molecular movement in a field of alternating electrical current at radiofrequency. An electromagnetic field is created around an active electrode when the frequency is set above 250 kHz. The active electrode is placed at the site for lesioning and an indifferent electrode is placed to minimize passage of current through the myocardium. Heat is generated in the tissues, which conducts to the active electrode. Heat is generated as current flows through a probe with a built in thermocouple needle. The heat is not emitted from the probe itself but from the current movement which generates the heat as it passes through the tissues. The lesion is formed once the neural temperature exceeds 45° C. Temperature above 90° C can cause boiling and tissue tearing with electrode removal. The temperature is monitored and wattage is adjusted to the desired level, which in turn determines the size of the lesion. Lesion plateaus with time. After 60 seconds at a certain temperature, lesion growth is minimal. The lesion is spheroidal and may extend several millimeters beyond the active electrode tip, but the majority of the lesion volume surrounds the axis of the active electrode. Prior to the lesioning, pain is first replicated using higher frequencies and lower voltages. Once the target tissue is localized, then only the thermocoagulation is instituted.

Technique proper: Once the needle or cannula position is perfectly placed at the desired site and level, the RF electrode is introduced via the cannula. With older systems, the electrode itself needed to be touching bone. With newer systems, utilizing a cannula sheathed with plastic or Teflon with an exposed metal tip of varying length, the electrode need not actually touch the bone, although the exposed tip must. Stimulation is then carried out, using a frequency of 50 Hz and a current up to 1 mA for sensory detection, and a frequency of 2 Hz with current between 3 to 5 mA for motor stimulation. A positive stimulation is that which reproduces the patient's pain, without producing other sensory or motor findings in the lower extremity or buttocks.

Negative stimulation may be failure to produce the patient's pain, or obvious stimulation of motor and sensory structures arising from the spinal nerve. In such cases, denervation should not be performed, and the cannula should be repositioned, followed by repeat stimulation.

Once the stimulation pattern is acceptable, a RF lesion is created by passing current through the electrode to raise the tissue temperature to 60 to 80° C for 60 to 90 seconds. This portion of the procedure may be quite uncomfortable, and judicious use of sedation and analgesics may be appropriate. Once the lesion is completed, the next level(s) can be treated in a similar fashion.

The usual complications encountered are as follows:
1. Neuritis/neuralgia – (Incidence -10%). Pain may be worse than the original pain.
2. Numbness; Motor paralysis.
3. Pneumothorax; Horner's syndrome.
4. Incomplete pain relief.

CONCLUSION

Chemical neurolysis or destruction of nerves either by the application of chemical neurolytic agents, which is an age-old accepted technique of achieving a pain relief in the chronic intractable pain patients, still continues to be one of the main armamentarium. Newer techniques like Radiofrequency lesioning and Cryoprobe have taken a front seat in the patient care recently and these are getting further improvized to produce effective prolonged analgesia for chronic pain syndromes. But, these techniques require specialized training, in depth knowledge of neural anatomy and understanding of chronic pain physiology. So, there application should be reserved only in painful conditions where conventional conservative pain management fails.

REFERENCES

1. Scholoesse. Heilung peripharer reizzustande sensibler and motorischer nerven klin Monatsbl Augenhilkd 1903;41:244.
2. Swetlow GI. Paravertebral alcohol block in cardiac pain. Am Heart J 1926;1; 393.
3. Digliotti AM. A new method of block anesthesia: Segmental peridural spinal anesthesia. Am J Surg 1933;20:107.
4. Arnott J. On the treatment of cancer by the regular application of an anesthetic temperature. London G Churchill 1851.
5. Smith LW, Fay T. Temperature factors in cancer and embryonal cell growth. JAMA 1939;113:60.
6. Labat G. Action of alcohol on the living nerve. Curr Res Anesth Analg 1933;12:190.
7. Myers RR, Powell HC. Galacose neuropathy: Impact of chronic endoneurial edema on the nerve blood flow. Ann Neurol 1984;16:587.

8. Gallagher HS, Yonezawa T, Hoy RC, Derrick WS. Subarachnoid alcohol block-II. Histological changes in the central nervous system. Am J Pathol 1961;35:679.

9. Mayo. Functional and histological effects of intraneural and intraganglionic injection of alcohol. Br Med J 1912;2:365.

10. Rumbsy MG, Finean JB. The action of the organic solvents on the myelin sheath of peripheral nerve tissue-II (short chain aliphatic alcohol). J Neurochem 1966;13:1509.

11. Myers RR, Katz J. Neural pathology of neurolytic and semidestructive agents. In Cousins MJ, Bridenbaugh PO (Eds). Neural blockade in clinical anesthesia and management of pain, (2nd Edn). Philadelphia, JB Lippincott 1988, 1031-1951.

12. Felsenthal G. Pharmacology of phenol in peripheral nerve blocks: A review. Arch Phys Med Rehabil 1974;55:13-16.

13. Smith MC. Histological findings following intrathecal injection of phenol solutions for the relief of pain. Anesthesia 1964;36:387.

14. Raj PP, Denson DD. Neurolytic Agents. In Raj PP (Ed): Clinical practice of regional anesthesia. New York, Churchill Livingston 1991.

15. Bonica JJ. Management of pain (2nd Ed.) Philadelphia, Lea and Febiger 1990, 1980-2039.

16. Lloyd JW, Barnard JDW, Glynn CJ. Cryoanalgesia, a new approach to pain relief Lancet 1976; 2:932-4.

17. Swerdlow M. Intrathecal neurolysis. Anaesthesia 1978; 33:733-40.

18. Paintal AS. Block of conduction in mammalian myelinated nerve fibers by low temperature. J Physiol 1965;180:1.

19. Myers RR, Powell HC, Costello ML, et al. Biophysical and pathologic effects of cryogenic nerve lesions. Ann neurol 1981;10:478.

20. Koning HM, Mackie DP. Percutaneous radiofrequency facet denervation in low back pain. The Pain Clinic 1994;7(3):199-204.

21. Sluijter ME. The use of radiofrequency lesions for pain relief in failed back patients. International Disability Studies 1988; 10(1): 37-42.

22. Wilkinson HA. Stereotactic radiofrequency sympathectomy. The Pain Clinic 1995; 8(1): 107-115

23. Shealy CN. Percutaneous radiofrequency denervation of spinal facets. J Neurosurgery 1975; 43:448-51.

24. Shealy CN. Facet denervation in the management of back and sciatic pain. Clin Orthop 1976; 115:157-64.

Section B

Documentation
and
Protocol

Four

Informed Consent for Interventional Pain Procedures

DK Baheti

Interventional procedure for treatment pain remains an important modality for relief of pain. All care is taken to make it simpler, free of stress and complications, cost effective however it is an invasive one so untoward effect or complications are unpredicted.

The scenario of practice of medicine has changed due to the internet explosion, medicolegal awareness and accountability. The information about the details of procedure to the patient and assuring him of successful outcome is necessary as we are dealing with a live person. The patient has every right to know the details of the procedure he is to undergo.

So it is mandatory for pain physician to inform the patient and his relatives the condition of patient, procedure to be performed its effects, outcome and unforeseen complications if any.

Following is the sample draft of informed consent form used by the author for interventional pain procedures, in more than 2000 pain relief procedures at Pain Management Clinic of Bombay Hospital and Medical Research Center and other centers nationally and internationally for more than fifteen years.

The same form is used by many pain physicians in India and abroad after obtaining the written consent from the author.

A word of caution for the pain physician who wants to use this form must check about the certain objectionable clause if any with notary or lawyer in their country.

Informed Consent for Pain Management Procedure Sample Form

Patient Name: _____

Age: _____ Sex: Male/Female   Date: _____

Address: _____

_____

I hereby authorize Dr. _____ to perform a Pain Management Procedure Known as _____.

This procedure has been explained to me by Dr._____ and I completely understand the nature and consequences of the said procedure. The following points have been made particularly clear.

1. Complications that may follow a procedure with/without relief of pain are same as those that may follow any other type of surgical procedure, such as infection, haematoma formation etc. These complications are enhanced in those cases where the patient is old and infirm, those with Diabetes and hypertension as also with those who have previous cardiac ailments and decompensation.

2. The drugs that are being used in this procedure are used generally in pain relief procedure alone. A patient may be allergic/idiosyncratic to this drug and may react to the drug in an unpredictable fashion and rarely with unpredictable results.

3. Rarely in some procedures may the procedure be followed with paralysis of one or more limbs? The risk of this has been explained to me.

4. In some procedures, specially prepared long needles have to be used. It is not always possible to use totally disposable needles in such cases. Though they are fully autoclaved the possibility of AIDS and B Virus hepatitis cannot be excluded.

5. Specially prepared needles are known sometimes, though rarely to break and if this happens a foreign body remains within the body and will require surgery to remove it. If such a procedure need be done then I permit Dr. _____ to get such operation performed a surgeon of his choice. Blood transfusions may be required during or after surgery. Though the blood is fully tested it may give rise to mismatch, B virus, Malaria as well as AIDS.

6. I understand that the Dr. _____ relies on the qualified staff provided by the hospital or nominated by him for postoperative care of the patient. He personally may not be able to visit the patient everyday.

I am aware that during the course of the procedure unforeseen condition may necessitate additional or different procedures that those set forth above. I therefore authorize and request that Dr.._____ to perform such procedures as are, in this professional judgment, necessary; these includes but are not limited to, procedures stated above. The

Authority granted therein, shall extend to remedying conditions that were unknown before the start of the operation.

I understand the risks of Local and General anaesthesia. I consent to the administration of anaesthesia under the supervision of Dr _____ or such anaesthesiologist that he shall select, and to the use of such anaesthesia as he may deem advisable.

The approximate recuperation time and the interval before I can return to work have been discussed with me. There is no guarantee when I shall be able to resume normal activities.

I consent to be photographed or filmed before, during and after treatment, and that these pictures will be property of Dr _____ and may be published inn scientific Journals and/or shown for scientific purpose.

I am known/not known allergic to any drug.

I agree to keep Dr. _____ informed of any change of address so that he can notify me of any late findings, and I agree to cooperate with Dr. _____ in the postoperative care until discharged.

I have read the above consent form/I have been explained the contents of this form in a language I understand _____ and I understand the contents.

I have had sufficient opportunity to discuss my condition with Dr. _____ and all my questions have been answered to my satisfaction. I believe that I have adequate knowledge on which to base an informed consent to the proposed treatment.

_____   _____
         Witness   Patient

I _____ (Relation _____) of the patient _____ have understood and been explained the contents of the above form. The patient cannot be explained as he/she is minor/is tense and can not be explained as he/she is mentally disturbed and I would rather sign the form.

_____   _____
         Witness   Relative

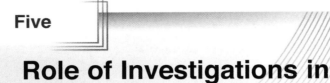

Five

Role of Investigations in Interventional Pain Procedures

DK Baheti

INTRODUCTION

Interventional procedure can lead to disturbances physiological and hemodynamic changes into the body, even though it is done with intention to relieve pain. It amounts to doing any surgical procedure. So it demands utmost care and precautions in order to make interventional procedure safe and can be repeated easily.

The investigations play an important role as it not only tells us about the physical condition of the patient but also leads to correct diagnosis of pain syndrome its management and therapy. However the investigation such as, imaging is a supplement to, not a substitute for a thorough history and physical examination.

Broadly investigations can be classified into biochemical and diagnostic.

Biochemical Investigations

Biochemical investigations are mainly laboratory investigations, such as:
1. Bleeding time, clotting time and INR: During Interventional procedure the needle can pass through any vessel and may lead to hematoma. Secondly many patients can be on thrombolytic agents such aspirin, clopedrogel, so it is vital to know the status of coagulation.
2. HIV and Australia Antigen.
3. Complete Blood Count: It will give us information about anemia and rise in white blood count indicate underlying infection.

Diagnostic

The diagnostic investigations are further classified as Imaging studies, Electromyography and Nerve conduction studies, Thermography,

IMAGING STUDIES

Imaging studies are Plane radiography, Computed tomography (CT), MRI, Myelography, Nuclear Medicine Scanning, Arthrography, and Discography.

The choice of modality depends upon tissue type and likely diagnosis. CT is best for severe, sudden headaches, trauma, and presumed sinusitis. MRI for chronic headache and temporomandibular joint dysfunction.

Plain Radiography (Figs 5.1 and 5.2)

It is very commonly available and least expensive modality and reliable one. It is rapid and portable. It gives the information about musculoskeletal disorders including trauma, abnormality of joints, bony structure, and osteophytes.

Computed Tomography (CT)

It will give us additional information of musculoskeletal system in compare to plain radiography, especially in regard to joint spaces. It is also helps in accurate placement of needle while celiac plexus block, cervical spine injections, and cranial nerve blocks.

Magnetic Resonance Imaging (MRI) (Figs 5.3 and 5.4)

It is modality of choice for spines to know the degree, position and extension of spinal cord compression due to protruding disc; Musculoskeletal, intracranial.

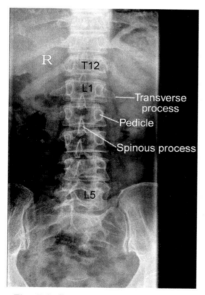 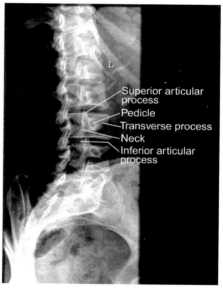

Fig. 5.1: Dorsolumbar spine-AP view   Fig. 5.2: Lateral view of lumbar spine

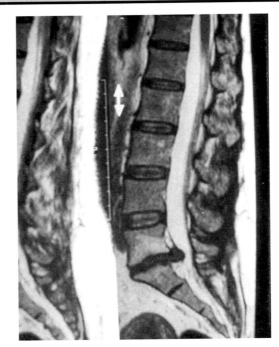

Fig. 5.3: MRI – showing disc protrusion at L5-S1

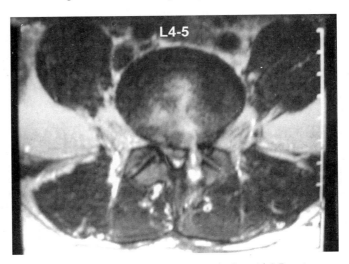

Fig. 5.4: MRI – showing root compression at L4-5 root

The use of Gadolinium contrast helps to identify early inflammatory and infectious process such as post-procedural discitis and suspected intrathecal catheter tip granuloma. The Gadolinium is iodine free, so it scores over other agents in iodine allergy patients.

MRI is contraindicated in ferromagnetic implants such as Cardiac pacemakers, intracranial clips or claustrophobic patients. One must verify with manufacturer for MRI compatibility, while performing intrathecal implants.

Myelography

This is done to visualize spinal canal and thecal sac. Nowadays MRI has replaced Myelography. However myelography is indicated in absence of MRI facility, where MRI does not correlate clinical findings and in claustrophobic patient.

Nuclear Medicine Scanning (Bone Scan) (Figs 5.5A and B)

This is bone scintigraphy with technetium (Tc)-99 phosphate. It indicates bone turn over in bone metastases and other disorders involving bone metabolism.

Arthrography

It is an injection of dye into joint space. Not very commonly done as, replaced by MRI.

Discography (Fig. 5.6)

This is done to localize the disc herniation or degeneration and for diagnostic purpose to know the cause of pain. It can be done in conjunction with CT

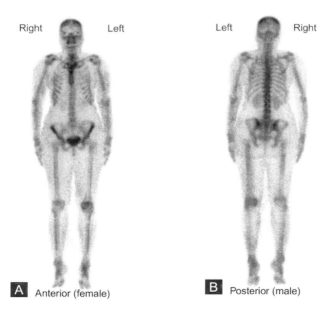

Figs 5.5A and B: Bone scan-Normal

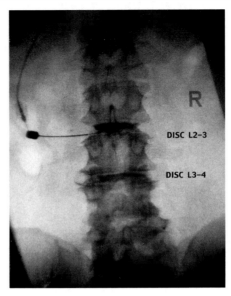

Fig. 5.6: Normal discogram- L2, 3

and MRI. Discography is invasive and has a risk of infection and neural injury so it should be used as confirmatory and not initially diagnostic tool.

Electromyelography (EMG) and Nerve Conduction Studies: Electrodiagnostic Studies (EDX) (Figs 5.7 and 5.8)

The history, symptoms, signs and physical examination is of prime importance. Any patient with neurological or muscular symptoms such as shooting or burning pain, numbness or weakness then EMG and Nerve conduction studies can be useful in the evaluation and treatment. Peripheral nervous system lesions such as dorsal root ganglion and distal can be assessed with these investigations.

In case of neuropathy EDX studies will show type of axonal or demyelinating; severity; as well as muscle involvement that may be present as a result of denervation of the muscle. Severe neuropathies may cause weakness.

The carpel tunnel syndrome may be bilateral, with only one hand clinically involved. So it is necessary to examine lower extremity as well to rule out generalized neuropathy.

For suspected neuropathies in tibialis anterior, EMG needle examination is recommended as it may show enervation. In order to confirm radiculopathies both EMG and Nerve conduction studies are necessary. As NCS may be normal, the needle EMG is diagnostic.

The temperature of extremity will significantly alter the nerve conduction studies.

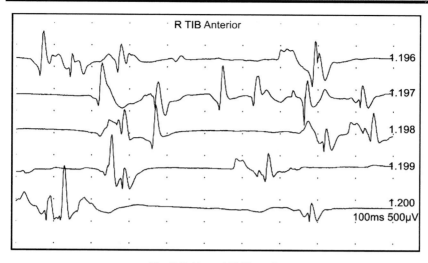

Fig. 5.7: Normal EMG tracings

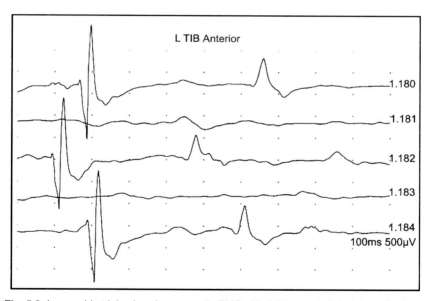

Fig. 5.8: Large wide triphasic units on needle EMG of Left TA muscle in Left L5 radiculopathy

In myasthenia gravis antibody assays are helpful to confirm the diagnosis.

The contraindication for EMG studies is uncooperative and unwilling patient, coagulopathies, lymph edema or anasarca and in patient muscle biopsy to be performed.

THERMOGRAPHY (FIG. 5.9)

Thermography is noninvasive procedure and easy to use. The qualitative data obtained reflect quantitative temperature difference up to 0.1°C. The examination room ambient temperature 20°C, carpeted floor, and examination table in center of room will give more precise information. The patient should wear light clothing, have not recently exercised, smoked, taken vasoconstrictor medicines.

Thermography is a sensitive tool to evaluate the dynamic physiological changes that reflect the underlying pathology. The changes in the pattern of temperature will help in differential diagnosis of pain due to peripheral nerve injury, spinal root pathology and CRPS. For example, increase in sympathetic activity causes vasoconstriction and resultant decrease in skin temperature. Whereas decreased sympathetic flow causes increase in regional blood flow which results in rise in skin temperature.

Thermographic images display temperature differentials in the entire area scanned. These images reflect alterations in blood flow superficially or up to 27 mm deep.

Colder temperatures are reflected as blue to black hues and warmer temperatures are pink to red. The difference in temperature provides important diagnostic information.

The mean temperature differential in peripheral nerve injury is 1.5°C. In sympathetic dysfunctions (RSD/SMP/CRPS) temperature differentials ranging from 1 to 10°C depending on severity are not uncommon. Rheumatologic processes generally appear as "hot areas" with increased temperature patterns. The pathology is generally an inflammatory process, i.e. synovitis of joints and tendon sheaths, epicondylitis, capsular and muscle injuries, etc.

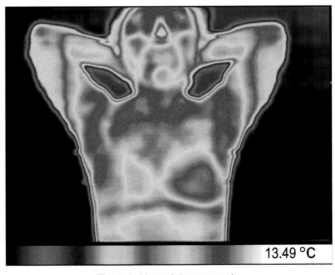

13.49 °C

Fig. 5.9: Normal thermography

Both hot and cold responses may coexist if the pain associated with an inflammatory focus excites an increase in sympathetic activity. Also, vascular conditions are readily demonstrated by DITI including Raynauds, Vasculitis, Limb Ischemia, DVT, etc.

RECOMMENDED FOR FURTHER READING

1. David Sutton- Textbook of Radiology

Six

Protocol for Interventional Pain Procedures: A Suggested Format

DK Baheti

An interventional pain procedure remains the main stay in the treatment protocol for relief of chronic pain and total pain management.

In the era of internet explosion the physician is accountable for his deeds while providing the pain relief procedure. In addition the insurance agency requires to be, satisfied before the reimbursement of the claim.

Hence it is mandatory for pain physician, to follow a strict protocol while performing any interventional procedure. It will not only provide the safety, minimum or no morbidity but also ensure the credibility of the procedure and so of the physician.

The suggested protocol is as follows:-

1. Complete evaluation and documentation of pain problem, history, symptoms, signs and investigations such as X-ray, CT Scan, MRI, Electromyelography, Nerve Conduction Study.
2. Explain the patient and family members about the procedure details, side effects, complications, if any.
3. Informed consent- must explain it in the language in which patient and his relatives understand, so they will sign the informed consent willingly.
4. Hospital admission for few hours to few days as the need be.
5. Investigations such as Bleeding time, clotting time, INR ratio (if patient on anticoagulants); HIV and Australia antigen.
6. Interventional pain procedure should be done either in operating room or procedure room equipped with monitoring and resuscitation facilities.
7. Pre procedure monitoring of Blood pressure, pulse.
8. Monitoring of the patient- Pulse, NIBP, and SaO_2.
9. Secure I.V. line.
10. I.V. antibiotic cover.
11. Sedation if necessary.
12. Anesthesiologist stands by as and when necessary.

13. Aseptic precaution such as wearing of gown, gloves, preparation of the area.
14. Lead gowns along with thyroid shield and radiation gloves (if possible) for all pain physician and lead gown for all staff present in procedure or operating room.
15. Radiation counter/measure monitor for pain physician.
16. Procedure tips
    A. Keep talking to the patient while performing the procedure, to allay the fear and anxiety.
    B. Follow rule of Three D's, i.e Direction, Depth, Destination while performing the procedure under fluoroscopy aim. Aim for Tunnel vision (Fig. 6.1).

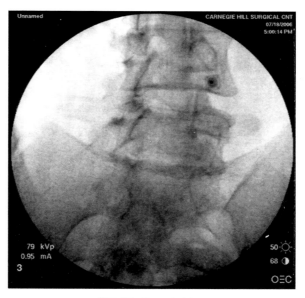

Fig. 6.1: Tunnel vision

    C. At regular interval push the needle about 1 cm and confirm the direction depth and destination.
    D. Repeated negative aspiration after confirming position of needle, injection of dye and local anesthetic agent, steroid, neurolytic agent.
    E. Confirm the spread of dye (Figs 6.2 and 6.3).

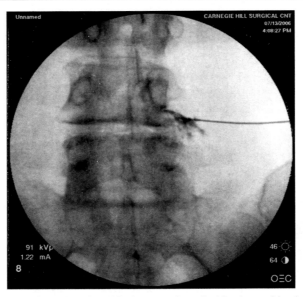

Fig. 6.2: Spread of dye- AP view-transforaminal lumbar epidural showing dye in epidural space with outlining of L4 nerve root sleeve

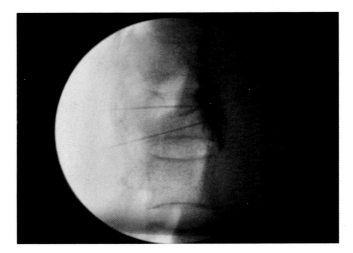

Fig. 6.3: Injection of dye and local anesthetic agent

F. Before injecting Neurolytic agent put gauze piece or abdominal sponge around the needle. This will prevent spilling of neurolytic agent on the skin and will prevent skin burns (Fig. 6.4).

G. Inject local anesthetic agent into the track of needle while withdrawing of the needle. This will reduce the post procedure pain at the site of insertion of needles.

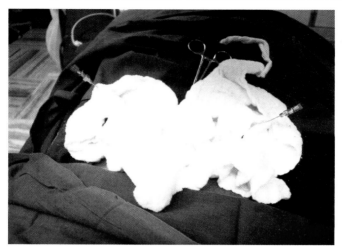

Fig. 6.4: Sponge around needles during celiac plexus block

17. Documentation in the form of print out, CD-one copy for record and one for patient.
18. Post-procedure monitoring of vital signs.
19. Follow-up advice must include
    • Dosage and schedule of medications
    • Explain about possible side effects of the drug
    • Date and time of next visit
    • Driving instruction to the patient if driving by himself.

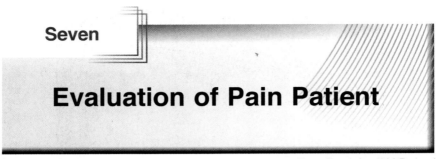

Seven

Evaluation of Pain Patient

Jitendra Jain, DK Baheti

Pain is one of the most fundamental symptoms of human species showing dysfunction of the body. Once Pain becomes chronic, it could get complicated. It might be then difficult to diagnose the physical or functional problem or the combination of both.

In recent years there has been tremendous interest in pain. As result of these modern researches there is a lot of information available about pain development at the Molecular, Physiological and Psychological level. As this information is applied in clinical practice more and more Clinicians are getting involved in the patient treatment. This is how Multidisciplinary Clinics are coming to picture.

Multidisciplinary clinics have clinicians from various specialities namely Pain Specialist, Neurologist, Psychiatrist, Spine specialist, General Physician, Physical therapist, Occupational therapist, Pain nurse, Social worker and Counselors and support staff. Depending on the availability specialist could be taken and group discussion could be held so as to give best of the multidisciplinary approach to the patient (Flow chart 7.1). Referring physician also plays an important role in alleviating patient anxiety about the Pain Clinic. He or she should be able to convince that the center is a pain centre where his problem would be heard and required treatment options would be suggested. Before these patients come to specialists for evaluation of the Pain, a Pain evaluation should be started by Pain nurse or the support staff.

Multidisciplinary Requirement

- Pain Physician
- Neurologist
- General Physician
- Psychiatrist
- Spine specialist
- Physical therapist
- Occupation therapist

- Psychotherapist
- Pain Nurse
- Social worker
- Support staff for clinic.

Flow chart 7.1: Showing approach to a pain patient with a multidisciplinary approach

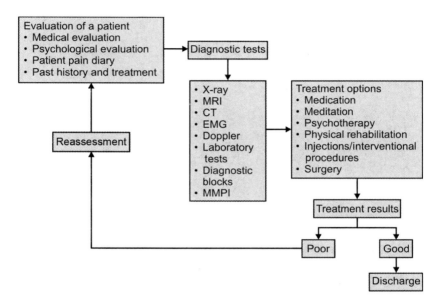

At our Clinic we have a team of specialist. Before patient comes to specialist he or she fills a pain evaluation form. It is actually a modified McGill Pain questionnaire with a local modification to suit patients and staff. It makes job of specialist very easy since almost all parts which could contribute to patient's pain are included in this form. Flow chart 7.1 is showing what should be a pain specialists approach for a pain patients which in reassessment in case of poor result. It is also important since it gives patient a sense of being heard and building rapport with the clinic. Patient should also explained about the steps of evaluation, i.e. after filling evaluation form there would be interaction with a clinician on the basis of evaluation form and examination and if required investigations. After all this treatment options would be suggested. It again helps patient gaining confidence about the clinician.

History

It is the most import part of patient management in pain. It gives us a full insight of patient, his problem, his expectation and possible treatment option.

General

It starts with knowing patient by name and calling him by his name. After this comes the contact details, age, sex, marital history, occupation, race, nationality and religion. Then one should start the pain history.

Chief Complain

What is the chief complain of the patient, e.g. is it Pain or Numbness. Because pain might have a treatment option but numbness might not have any treatment option. How did the pain start, trauma, accident or previous surgery, etc. one should note down VAS, i.e. Visual analogue scale of patients pain (Fig. 7.1).

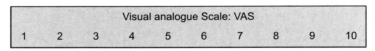

Fig. 7.1: Visual analogue scale

Pain History

History should revolve around pain, where, when, diurnal variation, severity, aggravating, relieving factors, referred pain patterns etc. A characteristic of pain is also important. It could be throbbing might indicate an inflammatory kind of a pain or a Burning pain which might indicate a neuropathic pain. Scary pain or fearful pain might give a hint about the patient personality and his tolerance to pain. Noting down these points is important since it helps in the treatment of the patient. Pain could be localized to one place might follow a nerve distribution or might even be diffuse. Every bit of information is important.

Pain Diagram

Pain diagram (Fig. 7.2) is the next important thing since it denotes the predominant pain site. If patients have pointed pain in virtually most of his body or back that might explain about the patient's mind and his or her expectation from a pain specialist. Also if in the second visit if patient's pain shifts from its original description might need a reassessment or gives us guide to send the patient to a psychotherapist for analysis.

Past Medical History

Patient's past medical history might indicate towards an accident or abuse or previous surgery which might help in treating the patient. Also what kind of treatment has the patient tried should be mentioned. Has he visited lots of doctors or hardly any is also helpful in devising treatment strategy. Associated medical illness which might be contributing to his pain needs to be attended.

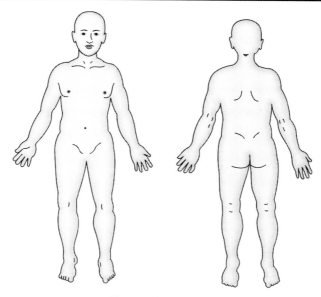

Fig. 7.2: Pain diagram

Family History

Health of family members, siblings' relations with them, disputes, family stress, divorce, financial problems or even abuse history might be helpful.

Personal History

Drug addiction, alcoholism, financial issues, social habits, behavior or sleep problems gives us an insight about patients pain problem.

Having all above information is important because it helps in understanding patients pain problem as well gives us an insight about his personality, his mental make up and expectations. For example, patients having pain all over body with numbness all over, giddiness and history of depression is less likely to respond to an interventional procedure than psychiatry counseling. History abuse in the patient in childhood or by the husband or a family member would also need counseling. Patient with a back pain who doesn't want surgery could be helped by interventional procedure. So one can do an overall assessment to see who would need what kind of treatment to start with.

Following questionnaire shows the General kind of Pain questionnaire. It mentions about what all kind of leading pain questions to be asked so as to get best information about patient's pain. VAS score is very important along with diurnal variation of pain. It also helps assessing improvement in patients since the first visit to the clinic. All the points mentioned in type of pain and disability could also be given score to get a better assessment.

Pain Questionnaire (smaller version)

PAIN QUESTIONNAIRE

GENERAL INFORMATION OF PATIENT: INCLUDING NAME, AGE, SEX, HEIGHT, WEIGHT, MARITAL STATUS, ALLERGIES, OCCUPATION, CHILDREN ETC.

PRESENT VAS SCORE: (VAS from 1-10)

PAIN DIAGRAM:

SITE, ONSET, DURATION AND PROGRESSION OF PAIN:

TYPE OF PAIN: THROBBING/SHOOTING/STABBING/BURNING/CRAMPCURRENT LIKE/ SHARP/ACHE/SPLITTING/SICKENING/FEARFUL/DEADLY/ EXHAUSTING

PAIN IN LAST 24 HRS:

PAIN DAIRY OR DIURNAL VARIATION OF PAIN:

AGGRAVATING FACTORS:

RELIEVING FACTORS:

CONTRIBUTING FACTORS:

DISABILITY:

- **PHYSICAL:** WALKING/SITTING/STANDING/SLEEPING/SEX/POSITION CHANGE
- **FUNCTIONAL:** MOOD SWING/CAN'T WORK OR PERFORM/NOT ENJOYING LIFE/ AFFECTING RELATIONS

ASSOCIATED PAIN OR REFERRED PAIN:

ANY INVESTIGATIONS:

ATTEMPTED TREATMENT: HOW LONG AND HOW EFFECTIVE

ASSOCIATED ILLNESS AND TREATMENT:

PERSONAL HISTORY: MARITAL/ ADDICTION/DRUGS/SLEEP/DEPRESSION OR OTHER SIGNIFICANT HISTORY

PAST HISTORY:

FAMILY HISTORY:

Examination

It is usually done to ascertain the cause of pain and its relation to the underlying disease. Even if it might not be really beneficial in some cases but still it assures about the competence level of the physician and he feels that his complains have been taken seriously. Patient should be appropriately undressed, if situation demands undress fully. It is advisable to have a female attendant with you while examining a female patient. Specific examination of various parts of body is beyond the scope of this chapter. Our attempt is to give you an overview of the examination so one does not neglect an important aspect of the examination.

General Examination

Built of the patient, skin color, weight loss signs, weakness, contractures, deformity, swelling of limbs and posture. Pulse, respiration, blood pressure, height and weight should be recorded while observing patient for signs of anxiety, tremors or sweating etc.

Systemic Examination

It is not always needed in depth unless patient has a systemic disease but is usually required to complete the list.

Localized Examination

One should be careful and warn patient of increased pain while performing localized area examination. If patient doesn't want that area to be touched then kindly make a note of it and report accordingly after inspection of the local area.

Inspection: It should involve checking the color of skin, surrounding area skin color, scar, wasting in comparison to opposite side, swelling or loss creases etc. also range of motion around that area or joint should be observed. Active and passive movement should be observed.

Palpation: It should include first palpating the painful area, is it tender or finding a trigger point, consistency feel, presence of allodynia or hyperesthesia etc. Palpating the surrounding area for pain is also important. Patient's reaction while examining him or her should be noted. Shouting or constant crying while examination indicates about the pain behavior of patient.

Neurological Examination

It is usually a must during examination. It might include cranial nerves if required otherwise usually include examining the area involved with the opposite side area or limb. In case of upper limb, lower limb examinations should be done to see if there is any lower limb involvement and vice versa.

Sensory: Pinprick, light touch, position sense, reflexes, strength and vibration of the dermatomes or an individual peripheral nerve.

Motor: Muscular atrophy, gait, power, flicker or flutter of localized muscles etc. of the group of muscles or individual muscle.

Cerebrum: Mood, Memory, Orientation etc.

Sympathetic Function: Sweating, Piloerection to gentle stroking of affected skin and Skin temperature.

Specific Examinations

Straight leg raising for Lumbar disc prolapse, spine flexion, extension and rotation with reporting of localized pain and its referring pattern. Breath related pain could be examined in trunk related cases. Specific area related examination is beyond the scope of this chapter but should be performed so as to come to a diagnosis.

Sometimes it might be difficult to perform examination due to extreme pain. Diverting patient's mind might sometimes decrease pain and allows examination. It should be tried in difficult cases. There is nothing in having a shorthand book of examination in the clinic so one can just browse through before or during examination.

Only after a thorough history and examination one should think of sending the patient for a laboratory investigation or a scan. One should not forget that patient's pain and laboratory report or scan finding might correlate. One must always record visual analogue scale of the patient during interview.

Diagnostic Evaluations

Depending on patient's history and examinations laboratory tests or scanning or X-rays are asked for. Depending on clinical impression patient might be even sent for a proper psychosocial evaluation. If required one might need to do a differential diagnostic interventional block like in cases of low back pain.

Commonly Done Diagnostic Tests

- X-ray of respective area.
- Scan either MRI or CT of the respective area. Sometimes it might needed to be done with contrast so as to enhance scanning as in cases of failed back surgery. Also in the patients with cancer pain to detect the spread.
- Doppler scan for limb pain.
- Bone scan for back or limb joints or metastasis.
- EMG and Nerve conduction studies.
- HLA B27, RA factor, ANA, Uric acid might be required to rule Immunological arthritic disorders.

  Still inspite of all above investigations one needs to correlate these finding with patients symptom and treat accordingly.

Diagnostic Tests

- Nerve root blocks to assess the level which is causing pain in cases of confusion about multiple levels
- Median branch block for Facet Syndrome
- Discography in cases with multiple levels Discogenic pain
- Sympathetic block to ascertain Sympathomimetic pain.

  These are few blocks mentioned are usually useful in cases where there is diagnostic dilemma inspite of scans etc. and Pain generator could not be found. Also before performing a Neurodestructive procedure a diagnostic block is a must. Depending on the pain generator, therapeutic modality needed to treat one particular pain could be applied so as to treat patients pain.

RECOMMENDED FOR FURTHER READING

1. Bonica's Management of Pain: (3rd Edn), Chief editor; John D Loeser. Lippincott Williams and Wilkins.
2. Melzack R. The McGill pain questionnaire: Major properties and scoring methods. Pain 1975;1:277-99.

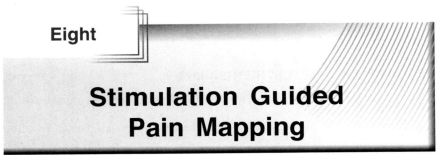

Eight

Stimulation Guided Pain Mapping

Sanjeeva Gupta, Jonathan Richardson

INTRODUCTION

Pain is a subjective symptom and expression of pain for the same degree of nociceptive input can vary between individuals. The nerve roots involved in carrying the nociceptive impulses can be identified either by looking at the pain dermatomal maps or by injection of a small amount of local anesthetic along the nerve roots involved and assessing the patient's response. There is always a possibility that the injected local anesthetic can soak adjacent nerve roots, which can confuse the issue. Stimulation guided steriotactic pain mapping allows us to identify precisely the nerve roots involved in carrying the nociceptive impulses and gives us an anatomical diagnosis of the nerve roots involved. This can help us to target the available treatments precisely. In our experience we have found this technique useful when patients complain of symptoms from a wide area of a particular part of the body.

Indications

The procedure is indicated when patients have pain in a particular part of the body and the nerve roots involved in carrying the nociceptive impulse needs to be identified to plan further management.

Contraindications

Absolute contraindications: Systemic or localized bacterial infection in the region of the block to be performed, bleeding diathesis, possible pregnancy. *Relative contraindications:* Allergy to contrast medium and local anesthetic.

Equipment

Fluoroscopy is mandatory: The procedure is performed under aseptic conditions. 25G and 21G hypodermic needles, 2ml and 5 ml syringes can be used.

Section C

Head and Neck

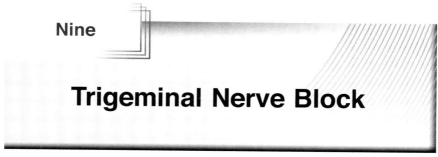

Nine

Trigeminal Nerve Block

Jitendra Jain

Trigeminal neuralgia (TN) is one of the classical neuropathic pain conditions that have been known for centuries.[1] As far as history is concerned, Absolute alcohol injection was first described by Hartel[2] then in 1965 Hakanson S[3] described Radiofrequency lesioning and Fujimaki T[4] about the Glycerol injection for the Trigeminal Neuralgia.

The International Association for the Study of Pain and the International Headache Society both have diagnostic criteria for trigeminal neuralgia (TN) that emphasize the severe paroxysmal nature of typical trigeminal neuralgia. The paroxysms of electric shock like pain that are often triggered by light mechanical stimulation of a trigger point are extremely painful. Treatment for it is initial pharmacotherapy with anticonvulsants like Carbamazepine, Gabapentine and the latest one Pregabalin. If the symptoms are not controlled by these medications or have side effects which are not tolerable then advanced option like Interventions by means of Neurolysis of Trigeminal nerve[5] or Thermocoagulation by Radiofrequency[6] current could be attempted as a minimally invasive safer option.

ANATOMY

Trigeminal nerve is one of the largest cranial nerves. It carries sensory fibers from Oral Mucosa, Conjunctiva, Tooth pulp, Gingiva and also anterior and middle cranial fossa. Trigeminal ganglion which is also known as Gasserian ganglion lies in Meckel's cave which is close to petrous part of temporal bone, it is formed by the two roots that exit the ventral surface of the brainstem at the mid pontine level. Meckel's cavity or cave lies in the middle cranial fossa. Medial to Trigeminal ganglion is bounded by the cavernous sinus; superiorly by the temporal bone of the brain and posteriorly is the brainstem. It gives off three branches intracranially namely—Ophthalmic, Maxillary and Mandibular. The exit of these three nerves is superior-medial to lateral and inferior respectively. Ophthalmic and Maxillary are sensory nerves while a small motor root joins mandibular division as it exits the cranial cavity via the foramen ovale (Figs 9.1 and 9.2).

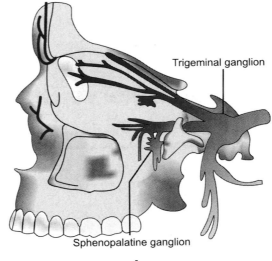

A

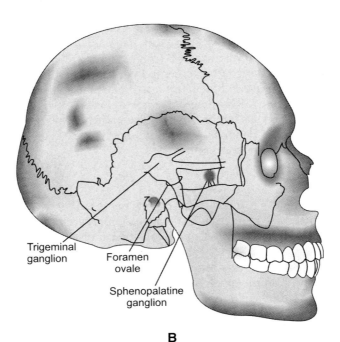

B

Figs 9.1A and B: Showing the trigeminal ganglion, its branches, foramen ovale and sphenopalatine ganglion

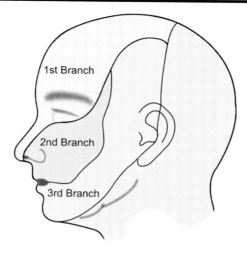

Fig. 9.2: Showing facial area cover by trigeminal nerve branches V1 (1st Ophthalmic), V2 (2nd Maxillary) and V3 (3rd Mandibular)

Indications

- Trigeminal neuralgia
- Cluster headache
- Intractable facial pain
- Oral or facial cancer
- Postintracranial or microvascular surgery pain
- Ocular pain due to glaucoma.

Contraindications

- Infection
- Sepsis
- Coagulopathy.

Equipment and Drugs

- 25G ¾ inch needle
- 22G 1½ inch needle or spinal needle
- 10 cm radiofrequency needle with 5 mm active tip
- 5 ml and 10 ml syringe
- 1 to 2% lignocaine
- 0.25 to 0.5% bupivacaine
- Depot steroids usually not required
- 6 to 10% phenol 1 ml
- Alcohol 95 to 97%
- Glycerol 40 to 50%
- Radiofrequency generator.

Preparation

Preprocedure history and physical examination of the local area before Trigeminal ganglion block is a must. Coagulation profile and requisite preoperative blood investigation of the patient could be done depending on the patient.

For this block usually sedation is required especially when Radio-frequency Thermocoagulation ablation is planned.

Patient is explained about the nature of the procedure. Patients is also informed that during the procedure he would be asked about numbness or current like sensation on face while stimulating the nerve and if it is covering the area of his pain. Patient should be told that there might be slight numbness over face after the procedure.

Position

Supine with extension of cervical spine and if needed roll under the shoulder blade, depending upon the C-arm visualization

Procedure

Preoperative antibiotic and intravenous sedation is supplemented before starting the procedure. Usually the entry point for the needle for Trigeminal block is 2.5 to 3 cm from the angle of the mouth. First antiseptic is applied. Local anesthetic using 1% Lignocaine is given along the skin and possible track of Radiofrequency needle but well short of foramen ovale with the spinal needle (Fig. 9.3).

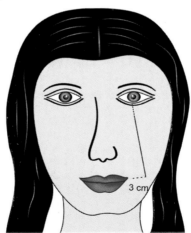

Fig. 9.3: Showing the direction of the needle, to be entering 2.5 to 3 cm from the angle of mouth and not medial to the center of the pupil

There are few different ways in which C-arm could be placed for doing Gasserian Ganglion block.

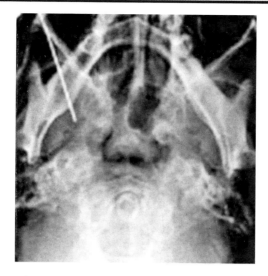

Fig. 9.4: Showing needle in the foramen ovale in submental view.
Also try to appreciate the foramen ovale on the opposite side

- Submental position of the face and jaw or of the beam of C-arm (Fig. 9.4).
- Caudal and lateral movement of C-arm so as to get the foramen between the mandibular ramus and maxillary sinus and foramen ovale is then visible as a slit opening usually near the upper half of Mandibular ramus
- Good old lateral C-arm placement while directing the needle into the foramen ovale (Figs 9.5 and 9.6).

In first two ways of placing C-arm the needle is directed towards the foramen ovale with "Tunnel view" and once deep enough and nearing foramen ovale lateral view is taken so as to check the depth of the needle. Once the needle enters foramen there might be sharp pain to patient as needle might be close to the mandibular nerve at the entry point of the foramen ovale. Needle is pushed till the intersection of petrous part of temporal bone and clivus. Needle should not be pushed beyond that point (Figs 9.5 and 9.6).

Confirmation is usually by C-arm. If required contrast with iopamide 0.1 ml or 0.5 ml could be injected. There might be CSF flow from needle. Most confirmatory would be stimulating the required segment of the nerve, either V1 or V2 (Maxillary) or V3 (Mandibular). V2 or V3 is more common than ophthalmic division, i.e. V1.

Neurolysis

Usually Glycerol is used for Neurolysis of the Gasserian Ganglion. Alcohol and Phenol Neurolysis is not recommended for trigeminal ganglion neurolysis. Contrast injection of iopamide checks the correct placement of needle and then Glycerol to about 0.1 to 0.5 ml is injected. Patient is warned

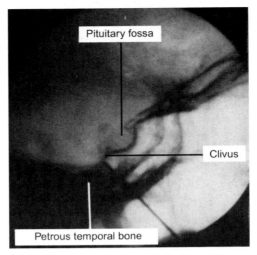

Fig. 9.5: Shows needle inside the foramen ovale in lateral C-arm view. Needle is just touching the clivus and not deeper than that, also approximately at the intersection of the clivus and petrous part of the temporal bone

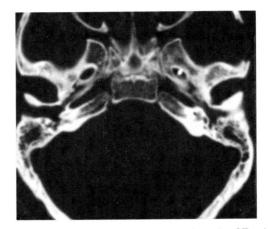

Fig. 9.6: Showing needle in the foramen ovale under CT guidance

of sudden pain or headache due to glycerol injection. Before injecting glycerol clear CSF flow is required and patient is place in semi sitting position with neck flexed for next 2 hours so that neurolysis of V2-V3 only occurs.

Radiofrequency Ablation

Trigeminal ganglion should get stimulated with sensory stimulation at 50 to 100 Hz with 0.1 to 0.5 V. Patient is asked to confirm the numbness or stimulation over face. Confirmation that numbness covers the painful area is the prerequisite before starting the Radiofrequency ablation. CSF leakage is not a must for Radiofrequency but negative aspiration with optimum impedance of 150 to 400Ω is desirable. After confirmation either good intravenous sedation or local anesthesia with 0.25% bupivacaine or 2% lignocaine at the trigeminal ganglion level is required so as to minimize the pain of Radiofrequency ablation. One has to make sure that there is no intracranial leakage before injecting local anesthetic.

Heating could be started at 46°C or at 55°C as test lesion then increase to about 60 to 70°C for 90 seconds. The conventional setting of 80°C for 60 sec to 90 sec is not recommended so as to decrease incidence of loss of corneal reflex and risk of anesthesia dolorosa. At least 2 lesions at that level would be giving a good Thermocoagulation near the ganglion level.

Pulsed Radiofrequency is a good option for Trigeminal neuralgia patients. The usual setting would be used, i.e. 42°C for 120 sec. again at least 2 cycles should be used. It would help preserve the corneal reflex and also decrease the incidence of anesthesia dolorosa. Although long-term results are doubtful but still it remains an attractive mode to be used for these patients.

Other minimally invasive interventional modalities used for Trigeminal Neuralgia Treatment:
- Microcompression lesioning
- Gamma Knife Radio-lesioning
- Permanent peripheral electrode stimulation.

Complications

- Anesthesia dolorosa
- Loss of corneal reflex
- Neurolytic keratitis
- Retrobulbar hematoma
- Carotid puncture
- Meningitis
- Intracranial brainstem radiofrequency lesioning
- Motor deficit of mandibular nerve, mastication difficulty
- Cheek hematoma.

Post-procedure it could be advisable to put ice pack over the cheek so as to decrease the cheek hematoma. Procedure is usually day care and patient could be discharged after few hours of the procedure unless the attending doctor feels otherwise.

If one is careful and observant with the point mentioned above for doing the procedure then one should not observe above listed complications. In case of V1 sensory deficit one should visit ophthalmologist regularly.

In most cases pain relief is immediate with immediate cessation of medication. Sometimes relief might take more than 1 to 2 week to be effective. These procedure are very effective with most patients have pain relief of usually more than their expected duration of pain relief, i.e. 6 months in case of radiofrequency ablation or even neurolysis. After recurrence procedure could easily be repeated. While performing repeat procedure one should be cautious as there might be fibrosis especially after neurolysis or difficult previous procedure of radiofrequency ablation. In older and edentulous patients the skin entry point could be made between 3 to 4 cm from the angle of the mouth so as to enter foramen ovale straight rather then at an angle.

REFERENCES

1. P Prithvi Raj, et al. Radiographic Imaging for Regional Anesthesia and Pain Management (1st edn). Churchill Livingston 2003.
2. Steven Waldman. Atlas of interventional pain management (2nd edn). Saunders 2004.
3. Håkanson S. Comparison of surgical treatments for trigeminal neuralgia: Re-evaluation of radiofrequency rhizotomy. Neurosurgery 1997;40:1106-7.
4. Fujimaki T, Fukushima T, Miyazaki S. Percutaneous retrogasserian glycerol injection in the management of trigeminal neuralgia: Long-term follow-up results. J Neurosurg 1990;73:212-6.
5. Fraioli B, Esposito V, Guidetti B, et al. Treatment of trigeminal neuralgia by thermocoagulation, glycerolization, and percutaneous compression of the gasserian ganglion and/or retrogasserian rootlets: Long-term results and therapeutic protocol. Neurosurgery 1989;24:239-45.
6. Taha JM, Tew JM, Buncher CR. A prospective 15-year follow up of 154 consecutive patients with trigeminal neuralgia treated by percutaneous stereotactic radiofrequency thermal rhizotomy. J Neurosurg 1995;83:989–93.

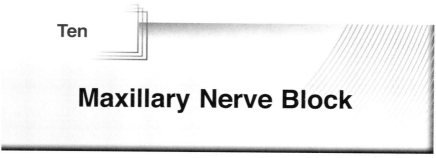

Ten

Maxillary Nerve Block

Jitendra Jain

INTRODUCTION

Maxillary nerve is the 2nd division of the Trigeminal nerve, also know as V2 division of Trigeminal nerve. Blocking of Maxillary nerve is useful for nasal, upper jaw pathologies.

ANATOMY (FIG. 10.1)

It is purely sensory nerve. As 2nd division of the Trigeminal Ganglion it goes anteriorly and inferiorly along the cavernous sinus through the foramen rotundum. It continues along the pterygopalatine fossa in the inferior portion of the infraorbital foramen. It is accompanied by the Maxillary artery in the

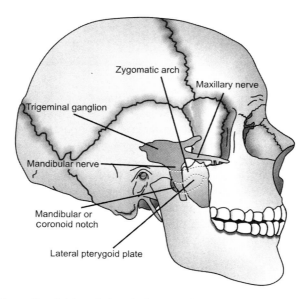

Fig. 10.1: Shows the division of trigeminal nerve. Maxillary nerve the V2 division travel just above the lateral pterygoid plate in the pterygopalatine fossa

pterygopalatine fossa. The sensory fibers connect the maxillary nerve to the sphenopalatine ganglion by way of five branches. Sensory branches of maxillary nerves which are about 10 in number carry sensation from soft palate, hard palate, gums, teeth, upper jaw, dura and parasympathetic fibers.

Indications

- Regional anesthesia for maxillofacial surgeries
- Diagnostic and therapeutic block for chronic nasal, upper jaw paiful conditions such as cancer.

Contraindications

- Local, nasal infection
- Coagulopathies
- Distorted anatomy.

Equipment and Drugs

- 25G ¾ inch needle, for local infiltration
- 22G 1½ inch needle or spinal needle, depending on the built of the patient
- 5 ml and 10 ml syringe
- 1 to 2% lignocaine
- 0.25 to 0.5% bupivacaine
- Depot steroids usually triamcinolone or alphamethyl prednisolone 40 mg
- 10 cm radiofrequency needle with 5 mm active tip
- Radiofrequency generator
- Alcohol 99%
- Phenol 6%.

Preparation

Preprocedure history and physical examination of the local area before maxillary nerve block is a must. Coagulation profile and requisite preoperative blood investigation of the patient could be done depending on the patient.

For this block usually no sedation is required unless radiofrequency thermocoagulation ablation is planned. Patient is explained about the nature of the procedure. Patients is also informed that during the procedure he or she might feel numbness or current like sensation in the nose or upper jaw when needle is maneuvered to target area or while stimulating the nerve. Patient should be told that there might be slight numbness over nasal, upper jaw area after the procedure.

Position

- Supine position or sitting if patient is co-operative with head straight looking at the ceiling.
- Make sure height is comfortable for you to do the block.

Procedure

Preoperative antibiotic is supplemented before starting the procedure. Usual external approach is from the center of the Coronoid notch, i.e. mandibular notch of the mandibular bone. Point of entry is just below the zygomatic arch and anterior to temporomandibular joint. First antiseptic is applied. Local anesthetic using 1% lignocaine is given along the skin. Needle is then pushed medially perpendicular to the skin. After about a distance of 3 to 5 cm one might encounter bone which would be lateral pterygoid plate of sphenoid bone (Figs 10.2 and 10.3). Once the lateral pterygoidal plate is hit then the needle is withdrawn and directed anterio-superiorly at about 45 degrees. One should go past the Lateral pterygoid plate. Needle should not go beyond 1.5 cm after hitting lateral pterygoid plate. Paresthesia might be encountered if maxillary nerve is hit. Use of peripheral nerve stimulator would be strongly recommended to place the needle as close to the maxillary nerve as possible. C-arm could also be used to reassure the placement of the needle by injecting contrast. Once confirmed the placement then 2 to 4 ml of local anesthetic is injected. If it is a diagnostic block then 1 to 3 ml is sufficient or else for a therapeutic block 3 to 5 ml is injected.

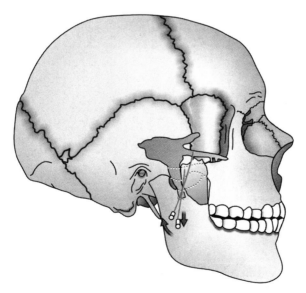

Fig. 10.2: Needle hits the lateral pterygoid plate and then is redirected towards maxillary nerve

Under C-arm guidance the needle is entered in the usual fashion and directed towards the inverted vas on the C-arm picture (Fig. 10.4A). Needle should not go further than lateral border of nose just at the superio-medial aspect of the maxillary sinus on the AP view of C-arm (Fig. 10.4B).

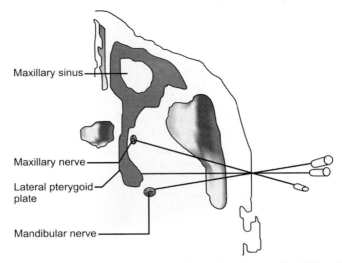

Fig. 10.3: Showing transverse section of the face showing needle hitting the lateral pterygoid plate and redirected for maxillary nerve. Also note needle direction for blocking mandibular nerve

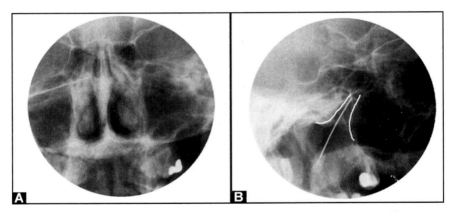

Figs 10.4A and B: Showing C-arm picture of needle placement for maxillary nerve block, A is in the lateral view and B is in the AP view

Neurolysis

Neurolysis is done for chronic pain maxillary, nasal, upper jaw, soft or hard palate cancers. Volume of the neurolytic solution should be same as the local anesthetic block, i.e. 3 to 5 ml. Neurolytic solution could be alcohol 99% or phenol 6%. It should be given slowly in 0.1 to 0.2 ml increaments so as to prevent accidental orbital, intracranial or vascular injection. One should keep in mind that as maxillary nerve is blocked in pterygopalatine fossa, sphenopalatine ganglion would also get blocked.

Radiofrequency Ablation

Radiofrequency ablation of the maxillary nerve is possible. Standard parameters should be for radiofrequency ablation of the maxillary nerve. Sensory stimulation of 50 Hz at 0.4 to 0.6 V would be the ideal response. Conventional radiofrequency is used at 80°C for 90 sec after injecting local anesthetic with 2 % lignocaine or 0.5% bupivacaine.

Pulsed Radiofrequency or Pulsed Electromagnetic field should be used for the peripheral nerve like maxillary nerve after confirming the needle placement. Lesion is made at 42°C for 120 sec. At least 2 to 3 lesions are done to a good pulsed radiofrequency lesion.

Complication

Usually maxillary nerve block is a very straight forward procedure if performed properly. Needle if pushed further could enter pterygomaxillary fissure. If pushed further could also enter orbit and block optic nerve as well leading to temporary or permanent blindness if neurolysis is done. Before injecting needle placement should be confirmed under C-arm guidance so as to prevent any accidental intravascular injection. There is also possibility of cheek hematoma.

RECOMMENDED FOR FURTHER READING

1. P Prithvi Raj, et al. Radiographic imaging for regional anaesthesia and pain management (1st Edn). Churchill Livingston 2003.
2. Steven Waldman. Atlas of interventional pain management (2nd Edn). Saunders 2004.
3. Romanoff M. Somatic nerve blocks of the head and neck. Raj PP. Practical management of pain (3rd Edn). St Louis, Mosby 2000;579-96.

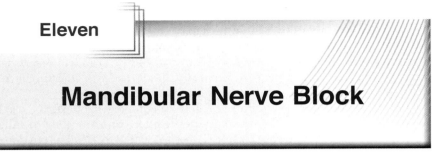

Eleven

Mandibular Nerve Block

Jitendra Jain

INTRODUCTION

Mandibular nerve is third branch of trigeminal nerve, known as V3 division of trigeminal nerve. Blocking of mandibular nerve is useful for post-operative pain relief of the jaw and also in chronic pain conditions like cancer of intraoral areas, e.g. lower jaw, tongue or oral mucosa, etc.

ANATOMY

Mandibular nerve emerges from the floor of middle cranial fossa.[1,2] As the V3 division of trigeminal nerve it comes out of the foramen ovale into the infratemporal fossa (Fig. 11.1). Infratemporal fossa where mandibular nerve

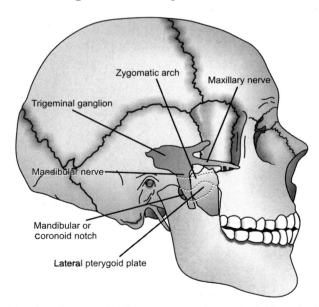

Fig. 11.1: Showing the mandibular nerve coming out of trigeminal nerve just posterior to the lateral pterygoid plate. Also shown in the diagram is the approach to the needle through the coronoid notch

enters after coming out of cranial cavity appears to be a rectangular structure. Posteriorly it is bound by the carotid sheath and styloid apparatus. Anteriorly is the posterior wall of the maxillary sinus, laterally is the ramus of mandible and medially it is bound by the lateral pterygoid plate which is the posterior extension of the sphenoid bone. It soon divides into small anterior and large posterior trunk. The small anterior trunk gives off branch to masseter the muscle of mastication and a sensory branch covering the sensory area overlying the muscle namely buccinator intraorally and over the skin.

The large posterior trunk divides into auriculotemporal, lingual and inferior alveolar nerve. It covers the anterior and external ear, temporomandibular joint, parotid gland and temporal area. Intraorally it takes sensory sensation from the anterior 2/3 of tongue, lower jaw and mucosa of the cheek.

Indications

- Chronic pain conditions like Ca. tongue, lower jaw or floor of the mouth
- Acute pain conditions like fracture of mandible, preoperative, intraoperative or postoperative conditions.

Contraindication

- Local infection
- Coagulopathies
- Distorted anatomy.

Equipment and Drugs

- 25G ¾ inch needle, for local infiltration
- 22G 1½ inch needle or spinal needle, depending on the built of the patient
- 5 ml and 10 ml syringe
- 1 to 2% lignocaine
- 0.25 to 0.5% bupivacaine
- Depot steroids usually triamcinolone or alphamethyl prednisolone 40 mg
- 10 cm radiofrequency needle with 5 mm active tip
- Radiofrequency generator
- Alcohol 99%
- Phenol 6%.

Preparation

Preprocedure history and physical examination of the local area before Mandibular nerve block is a must. Coagulation profile and requisite preoperative blood investigation of the patient could be done depending on the patient.

For this block usually no sedation is required unless Radiofrequency Thermocoagulation ablation is planned. Patient is explained about the nature of the procedure. Patient is also informed that during the procedure he or she might feel numbness or current like sensation on the jaw when needle is maneuver to target area or while stimulating the nerve. Patient should be told that there might be slight numbness over jaw area after the procedure. Also if neurolysis is planned then there might be weakeness in chewing from that side of the jaw.

Position

- Supine position or sitting if patient is cooperative with head looking at the ceiling
- Make sure height is comfortable for you to do the block.

Procedure

Preoperative antibiotic is supplemented before starting the procedure. Usual external approach is from the center of the coronoid notch, i.e. mandibular notch of the mandibular bone. Point of entry is just below the zygomatic arch and anterior to temporomandibular joint. First antiseptic is applied. Local anesthetic using 1% lignocaine is given along the skin. Needle is then pushed medially perpendicular to the skin. After about a distance of 3 to 5 cm one might encounter bone which would be lateral pterygoid plate of sphenoid bone (Figs 11.2 and 11.3). One needs to slowly walk past the posterior edge of the lateral pterygoid plate maintaining the same depth at the same level. Patient might encounter paresthesia at this point. Use of peripheral nerve

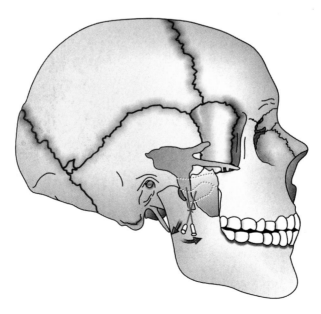

Fig. 11.2: Showing needle hitting the lateral pterygoid plate and redirected posteriorly to the mandibular nerve

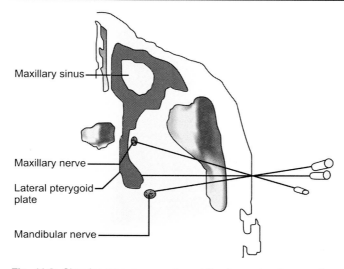

Fig. 11.3: Showing tranverse section of the face, showing needle hitting the lateral pterygoid plate and redirected for mandibular nerve. Also note that for blocking maxillary needle goes anteriorly

stimulator would be strongly recommended to place the needle as close to the nerve as possible. C-arm could also be used to reassure the placement of the needle by injecting contrast and using peripheral nerve stimulator. Once confirmed the placement then 2 to 4 ml of local anesthetic is injected. Continuous catheter could also be placed once the placement is confirmed especially for post-operative pain relief patients.

Neurolysis

Neurolysis is done for inoperable oral cancer patients, although it is not done very commonly. Volume of the neurolytic solution should be same as the local anesthetic block, i.e. 2 to 4 ml. Neurolytic solution could be alcohol 99% or phenol 6%. It should be used in incremental doses of 0.1 to 0.2 ml so as to prevent any form of accidental intravascular or intracranial injection.

Radiofrequency Ablation

Radiofrequency ablation of the mandibular nerve can be done instead of neurolysis. Standard parameters should be for radiofrequency ablation of the Mandibular nerve. Sensory stimulation of 50 Hz at 0.4 to 0.6 V would be the ideal response. Conventional radiofrequency is used at 80°C for 90 sec after injecting local with 2 % lignocaine or 0.5% bupivacaine.

Pulsed radiofrequency or pulsed electromagnetic field should be applied instead of conventional high temperature radiofrequency ablation after confirming needle placement. Lesion is done at 42°C for 120 sec. At least

2 to 3 lesions are done to a good pulsed radiofrequency lesion. Pulsed radiofrequency is strongly recommended instead of conventional high temperature (80°C) radiofrequency ablation so as to preserve the motor function. Immediate post-procedure there might be weakness of the jaw along with numbness. Patients should be warned about these in advance.

Complication

Usually mandibular nerve is a very straight forward procedure if performed properly. Needle if pushed further could enter pharynx. Needle could be close to middle meningeal artery in the infratemporal fossa. So careful aspiration is a must. Hematoma of the cheek is also a possibility.

Depth required to get the mandibular nerve should not be more than 5 to 6 cm. If one needs to go further kindly check the landmarks again used to do the block.

RECOMMENDED READING

1. P Prithvi Raj, et al. Radiographic imaging for regional anaesthesia and pain management (1st Edn). Churchill Livingston 2003.
2. Steven Waldman. Atlas of interventional pain management (2nd Edn). Saunders 2004.
3. Romanoff M. Somatic nerve blocks of the head and neck. Raj PP. Practical management of pain (3rd Edn). St Louis, Mosby 2000, 579-96.

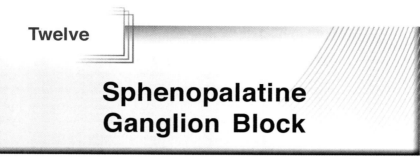

Twelve

Sphenopalatine Ganglion Block

Jitendra Jain

Sphenopalatine ganglion has generated interest of most of the medical faculty for various reasons. It has been blamed for facial pain, headache, dysmenorrhea, allergies and also sciatica.

ANATOMY (FIG. 12.1)

It is the largest group of neurons outside the cranial cavity. The SPG is one of four parasympathetic ganglia in the head. It is located in the pterygo-palatine fossa, posterior to the middle nasal turbinate under a 1 to 1.5 mm layer of connective tissue and mucous membrane and anterior to the pterygoid canal. This superficial location allows the block to be performed with topical anesthetic or by injection.

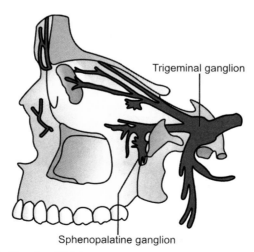

Fig. 12.1: Showing SPG in pterygopalatine fossa with suspended from maxillary nerve via sphenopalatine nerves

The pterygopalatine fossa is 1 cm wide and 2 cm high. It is bordered anteriorly by the posterior wall of maxillary sinus, posteriorly by the medial plate of the pterygoid sinus. Medially it has perpendicular plate of the palatine bone while laterally there is infratemporal fossa. Superiorly it has sphenoid sinus. Caudally the ganglion connects to the greater and lesser palatine nerve.

The sensory afferent axons traveling through the SPG arise from the maxillary division of the trigeminal nerve, which enters the pterygopalatine fossa through the foramen rotundum to lie just superior to the SPG. The sensory fibers connect the maxillary nerve to the SPG by way of five branches that extend from the nasopharynx, nasal cavity, palate, and orbit. The pharyngeal branch supplies the sphenoidal sinus and the mucosa of the roof of the pharynx via the palatine canal, the greater palatine nerves extend posteriorly, and the inferior nasal branches supply the palate via the greater palatine foramen. The tonsil and soft palate are supplied via the lesser palatine nerve as it arises from the lesser palatine foramen. The nasopalatine nerve emerges through the sphenopalatine foramen, passes along the nasal septum, and emerges through the median incisive foramen to reach the hard palate. The posteriorly is ethmoidal and sphenoidal sinuses below the periosteum of the orbit are supplied via the orbital branches. The nasal cavity is supplied via the posterior superior nasal branches.

Sphenopalatine ganglion has a very complex ganglion in terms of its neural connections. The nerve fibers leading into the SPG, i.e. sphenopalatine ganglion has sensory nerve supply via the sphenopalatine nerve and the maxillary nerve (establishing a strong "fine-fiber" connection between trigeminal fibers and parasympathetic fibers inside the ganglion). It also has the parasympathetic connection from the vagus nerve and the 3 vagal ganglia in the brain stem. Parasympathetic nerves travels on to the nucleus petrosus major and fibers of the facial nerve originating at the ganglia geniculi (establishing a connection to the 7th cranial nerve) which synapse in the SPG with postganglionic fibers. These postganglionic fibers go to the nasal mucosa and lacrimal glands.

The sympathetic connection is via the nucleus petrosus profundus (establishing a connection with the superior cervical ganglion and the SNS). The postganglionic fibers from upper cervical sympathetic ganglion join the carotid plexus. Then from there via deep petrosal nerves and vidian nerve they join the SPG.

Indications

- Sphenopalatine neuralgia
- Cluster headache
- Migraine
- Trigeminal neuralgia
- Atypical facial pain
- Post herpetic neuralgia of face
- Cancer pain of palate, base of tongue or pharynx.

Contraindications

- Local infection
- Coagulopathy.

Equipment and Drugs

- 25G ¾ inch needle
- 22G 1½ inch needle or spinal needle
- 10 cm radiofrequency needle with 5 mm active tip
- 5 ml and 10 ml syringe
- 1 to 2% lignocaine
- 0.25 to 0.5% bupivacaine
- Lopamide/Iohexol
- Methylprednisolone or triamcinolone diacetate
- Radiofrequency generator.

Preparation

Patient preparation for a sphenopalatine ganglion blockade consists of thorough patient education of the procedure, risks, benefits, expected outcome, written informed consent, and large bore intravenous access. Patient monitoring should include blood pressure and heart rate monitoring and pulse oximetry is advised to observe any potential cardiac effects. Ruling out local infection is a must. Radiofrequency ablation of SPG should be performed under sedation.

Position

Position of the patient is supine. C-arm is place in lateral position so that TM joint and external auditory meatus of both sides are overlap each other. Pterygopalatine fossa should be visible as "inverted vas" posterior to maxillary sinus and just anterior to anterior end of petrous part of temporal bone (Figs 12.2 and 12.3).

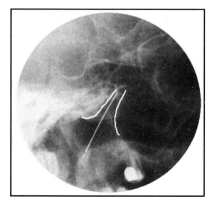

Fig. 12.2: Showing needle in the "inverted vas" under C-arm which is pterygopalatine fossa

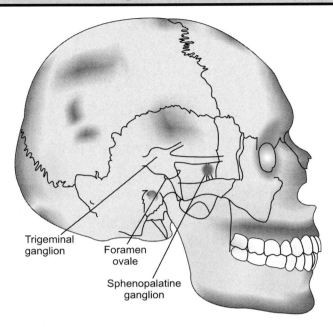

Fig. 12.3: Showing needle through the center of the coronoid notch, although in diagram it looks as if it is over zygomatic arch but in reality it goes underneath the zygomatic arch

Procedure

Under strict aseptic precaution the local anesthetic is injected under zygoma and above the coronoid notch. The radiofrequency insulated 10 cm needle is then inserted with its direction towards the inverted vas means slightly superior medial and anterior. Depth of the needle is checked on AP view. It should not cross the lateral border of nose and should sort rest at the superior-medial end of the maxillary sinus on C-arm (Fig. 12.4).

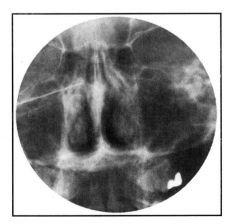

Fig. 12.4: Showing needle till the lateral border of nose and at the superior-medial end of maxillary sinus on the C-arm

Once the needle has reached the required area then stellate is removed and local anesthetic either bupivacaine 0.5% is injected or lignocaine 2% is injected with or without steroid. Volume usually should not be more than 2 ml, so if one is injecting contrast then be sure about the volume. Negative aspiration is must to blood or clear fluid which could even be CSF. This would mainly work as a diagnostic cum therapeutic block. If it is positive then radiofrequency of the same could be planned at a later date.

Radiofrequency Ablation[1,2]

Once the needle is in place then SPG is stimulated to 50 Hz at 0.4 to 0.6 V. Stimulatory response of the patient is important. If it stimulated upper teeth then one might be close the maxillary nerve. If one is having numbness or stimulation of hard or soft palate then needle might be inferior. The best stimulation felt is in the nose or at the base of the nose. Also there might be stimulation of the painful area. Once the stimulatory parameters are met then conventional radiofrequency is used at 80°C for 90 sec after injecting local with 2% lignocaine or 0.5% bupivacaine.

Pulsed radiofrequency or pulsed electromagnetic field could be applied as well once confirming the needle placement at 42°C for 120 sec. At least 2 to 3 lesions are done so get a good effective lesion of SPG.

Complications

- Bleeding as nose is rich in vasculature, usually respond to pressure
- Infection if nasal mucosa is breached at the lateral border of nose
- Bradycardia while performing radiofrequency ablation. Atropine should be kept ready.

After procedure patient might have hypoesthesia of palate, maxilla and of posterior pharynx. It is again a day care procedure and patient can go home after few hours of the procedure. In case of recurrence procedure could be easily repeated.

REFERENCES

1. Salar G, Ori C, Iob I. Percutaneous thermocoagulation for sphenopalatine ganglion neuralgia. Acta Neurochir (Wien) 1987;84:24-8.
2. Miles Day. Neurolysis of trigeminal and sphenopalatine ganglion: Pain practice 2001;1(2):171-82.

RECOMMENDED FOR FURTHER READING

1. Prithvi Raj, et al. Radiographic imaging for regional anaesthesia and pain management (1st Edn). Churchill Livingston 2003.
2. Steven Waldman. Atlas of interventional pain management (2nd Edn). Saunders 2004.

Thirteen

Glossopharyngeal Nerve Block

PN Jain

INTRODUCTION

Pain in the afferent distribution of the glossopharyngeal and vagus nerves may be felt in the larynx, base of the tongue, tonsillar region, ear and occasionally ipsilateral face, neck or scalp. Paroxysm of pain of unknown etiology occurring in this distribution may be due to glossopharyngeal neuralgia. The attacks are usually described as stabbing, sharp, 'like a knife', 'like an electric shock', and sometimes hot or burning. The intensity is probably less intense than trigeminal neuralgia (TN). It may indeed be confused with TN. Both neuralgias may be due to focal pressure along the course of the nerve. It may be tortuous vertebral artery or posterior inferior cerebellar artery impinging on the roots of ninth nerve. It may be trauma, local infection, alongated styloid process or ossified styloid ligament. However unlike TN, ninth nerve neuralgia is almost never associated with multiple sclerosis. Patients are often more than 20 years old. Men and women are equally affected. There is slight predominance of left sided cases in large series. Individual attacks commonly last seconds or minutes and rarely occurs at night. Pain is triggered by swallowing, yawning, coughing, and chewing. A variety of cardiovascular and other symptoms may accompany the attacks. Due to overlap of the sensory teritories of the seventh, ninth and tenth cranial nerves a lesion of one does not always cause loss of sensation in the throat or ear.

APPLIED ANATOMY (FIG. 13.1)

The glossopharyngeal nerve contains both motor and sensory fibers. The motor fibers innervate the stylopharyngeus muscle. The sensory portion of the nerve innervates the posterior third of the tongue, palatine tonsils, and the mucous membranes of the mouth and pharynx. Special visceral afferent sensory fibers transmit informations from the taste bud of the posterior third of the tongue. Information from the carotid sinus and body that helps control blood pressure, pulse and respiration is carried via the carotid sinus nerve which is branch of the glossopharyngeal nerve. Parasympathetic fibers pass

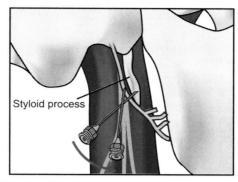

Styloid process

Fig. 13.1: Extraoral technique of IX nerve block

via the glossopharyngeal nerve to the otic ganglion. Postganglionic fibers form the ganglion carry secretory information to the parotid gland.

The glossopharyngeal nerve exit from the jugular foramen in proximity to the vagus, accessory nerves and the internal jugular vein. All three nerves lie in the groove between the internal jugular vein and the internal carotid during glossopharyngeal nerve block can result in intravascular injection or hematoma formation. Even small amounts of local anesthetic injected into the carotid artery at this location can produce profound local anesthetic toxicity (Fig. 13.2).

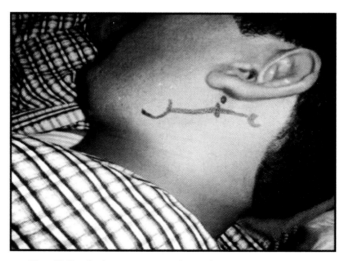

Fig. 13.2: Surface anatomy: glossopharyngeal nerve block

The landmarks for glossopharyngeal nerve block include the styloid process of the temporal bone. This osseous process represents the calcification of the cephalad end of the stylohyoid ligament. Although the process is usually easy to identify, if ossification is limited, it may be difficult to locate with the exploring needle.

Glossopharyngeal nerve block with local anesthetic may be utilized for palliation in acute pain emergencies, including glossopharyngeal neuralgia[1] and cancer pain, during the wait for pharmacologic, surgical, or anti-neoplastic methods to become effective. Additionally, this technique is of value in patients with atypical facial pain[2] in the distribution of the glosso-pharyngeal nerve. Glossopharyngeal nerve block[3] is also useful as an adjunct to awake endotracheal intubation.

Destruction of the glossopharyngeal nerve[4] is indicated in the palliation for cancer pain, for example, from invasive tumors of the posterior tongue, hypopharynx, and tonsils. The technique is also useful in the management of the pain of glossopharyngeal neuralgia that has not responded to medical management or in patients who are not candidates for surgical microvascular decompression.

Indications for glossopharyngeal Nerve Block

Local anesthetic block	Surgical anesthesia
	Prognostic block before neurolytics
	Adjunct to awake endotracheal intubation
Neurolytic block	Palliation of cancer pain
	Management of glossopharyngeal neuralgia

Contraindications to Glossopharyngeal Nerve Block

- Local infection
- Sepsis
- Coagulopathy
- Disulfiram therapy (if alcohol is used)
- Significant behavioral abnormalities

Local infection and sepsis represent absolute contraindications to all procedures. Coagulopathy is a strong contraindication for glossopharyngeal nerve block; however, owing to the desperation of many patients suffering from aggressively invasive head and face malignancies, ethical and humanitarian considerations dictate the use of this procedure despite the risk of bleeding.

If there are strong clinical indications, blockade of the glossopharyngeal nerve utilizing a 25-gauge needle may be carried out in the presence of coagulopathy, albeit with an increased risk of ecchymosis and hematoma formation.

TECHNIQUE OF GLOSSOPHARYNGEAL NERVE BLOCK

The Extraoral Approach

The patient is placed in the supine position. An imaginary line is visualized running from the mastoid process to the angle of mandible. The styloid process should lie just below the midpoint of this line. The skin is prepared with antiseptic solution. A 22-gauge, 1.5 inch needle attached to a 10 ml syringe is advanced through this midpoint location in a plane perpendicular to the skin. The styloid process should be encountered within 3 cm after contact is made the needle is withdrawn and "walked off" the styloid process posteriorly. As soon as bony contact is lost, and if careful aspiration reveals no blood or cerebrospinal fluid, 7 mL of 0.5% preservative-free lidocaine combined with 80 mg of methylprednisolone injected in incremental doses. Subsequent daily nerve blocks are carried out in a similar manner, substituting 40 mg of methylprednisolone for the initial 80 mg dose. This approach may also be utilized for breakthrough pain in patients who previously experienced adequate pain control with oral medications.

The Intraoral Approach

The tongue is anesthetized with 2.0% viscous lidocaine. The patient is asked to open the mouth widely, and the tongue is retracted inferiorly with a tongue depressor or laryngoscope blade. A 22-gauge, 3.5 inch spinal needle that has been bent about 25 degrees from horizontal is inserted through the mucosa at the lower lateral portion of the posterior tonsillar pillar. The needle is advanced approximately 0.5 cm after careful aspiration for blood and cerebrospinal fluid, local anesthetic or steroid is injected as for the extraoral approached glossopharyngeal nerve block.[5]

POTENTIAL COMPLICATIONS

The complications and unwanted side effects of blockade of the glossopharyngeal nerve blocked are as follows:
- Dysphagia
- Ecchymosis and hematoma
- Post-procedure dysesthesias, including anesthesia dolorosa
- Weakness of trapezius muscle
- Weakness of tongue
- Hoarseness
- Infection
- Tachycardia
- Local anesthetic toxicity
- Trauma to nerves
- Sloughing of skin and subcutaneous tissue.

The major complications are related to trauma of the internal jugular and carotid arteries. Hematoma formation and intravascular injection of local anesthetic with subsequent toxicity represent significant problems for the patient. Blocked of the motor portion of the glossopharyngeal nerve can result in dysphagia secondary to weakness of the stylopharyngeus muscle. If the vagus nerve is inadvertently blocked as often happens during glossopharyngeal nerve block, dysphonia secondary to paralysis of the ipsilateral vocal cord may occur. A reflex tachycardia secondary to vagal nerve block is also observed in some patients. Inadvertent block of the hypoglossal and spinal accessory nerves during glossopharyngeal nerve block results in weakness of the tongue and trapezius muscle.

A small proportion of patients who undergo chemical neurolysis or neurodestructive of the glossopharyngeal nerve experiences post-procedure dysesthesias in the area of anesthesia. These symptoms range from mildly uncomfortable burning or pulling sensation to severe pain. Severe post-procedure pain, called anesthesia dolorosa, can be worse than the patient's original pain complaint and is often harder to treat. Sloughing of skin and subcutaneous tissue had been associated with anesthesia dolorosa.

As mentioned previously, the glossopharyngeal nerve is susceptible to trauma from needle, hematoma, and compression during injection procedures. These complications, although usually transitory, can be quite upsetting to the patient.

NEURODESTRUCTIVE PROCEDURES

The injection of small quantities of alcohol, phenol, and glycerol into the area of the glossopharyngeal nerve has been shown to provide long-term relief for patients with glossopharyngeal neuralgia or cancer-related pain that has not responded to optimal trials of the previously mentioned therapies. Destruction of the glossopharyngeal nerve can be also carried out by creating a radiofrequency lesion[6] under biplanar fluoroscopic guidance. This procedure is reserved for cases that have failed all the previously described treatments for intractable glossopharyngeal neuralgia and in patients whose physical status precludes more invasive neurosurgical treatments.

REFERENCES

1. Dany JB. A study of four cases of glossopharyngeal neuralgia: Its diagnosis and treatment. Arch Sug 1927;15:198-215.
2. Walman SD. The role of neural blockade in the management of headaches and facial pain. Headache Digest 1991;4:286-92.
3. Brown DL. Glossopharyngeal nerve block. In Brown DL (Ed): Atlas of regional anaesthesia. Philadelphia, Lea and Febiger 1990;1996-9.
4. Waldman SD, Waldman KA. The diagnosis and treatment of glossopharyngeal Neuralgia. Am J Pain Management 1995;5:19-24.
5. Katz J. Glossopharyngeal nerve block. In Katz (Ed). Atlas of regional anaesthesia. Norwalk. CT. Appleton and Lange 1994:52.
6. Arbit E, Krol G. Percutaneous radiofrequency neurolysis guided by computerized tomography for the treatment of glossopharyngeal neuralgia. Neurosurgery.

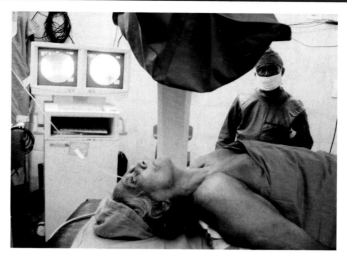

Fig. 14.4: Position for doing [R] stellate ganglion block

for blind approach. The jaw may be kept slightly open to relax the muscle. The patient should refrain from speaking as this can move the muscle and dislodge the needle. She should be instructed to raise his hand to indicate any difficulty.

The skin is aseptically prepared and draped. Index finger of the nondominant hand should be used for palpation of the landmarks. After making a skin wheal, 22 G short-bevel needle is introduced with the dominant hand directly posterior perpendicular to the table in all directions. The needle passes through underlying tissues till it contacts the bone at the C6 tubercle on transverse process or its junction with the vertebral body. Once the bone is encountered the needle is withdrawn 2 to 5 mm to avoid injecting into the longus colli muscle. The needle should preferably be attached to the extension tubing with the three-way to avoid chances of displacement while attaching the syringe. One can also release the dominant hand to aspirate and/or inject while grasping the hub with an artery forceps.

After negative aspiration, 2 to 3 ml of the dye can be injected to ascertain proper position of the needle tip. Aim for a linear spread of the dye in vertical direction on fluoroscopy (Fig. 14.5A). One can also verify the dye spread on lateral view (Fig. 14.5B). An initial test dose should be injected in all patients. An intravenous bolus of as less as 1.0 ml can produce seizure or loss of consciousness. Careful and repeated aspiration for CSF and blood is mandatory.

A modification of this technique includes needle placement at the C7 level.[7] This is impossible without imaging as there is no tubercle and injury to the pleura and vertebral artery is quite likely. The advantage is one can use minimal amount of the drug like 1 to 2 ml for sympathetic block of the head, face and neck.10 ml of local anesthetic is required to reach a level of T2/T3 to block sympathetic outflow of the upper extremity.[4]

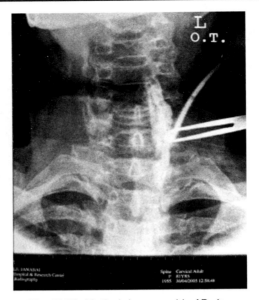

Fig. 14.5A: Vertical dye spread in AP view

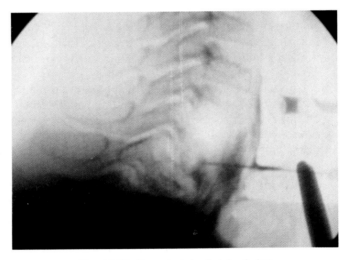

Fig. 14.5B: Spread of dye in lateral view

A continuous technique has been described where a thin Teflon catheter is inserted under image guidance onto C6 or C7 through a thicker cannula which is later on removed.[7] There is however a small risk of catheter migration to the dural cuff or adjacent vessels. A continuous infusion can be given to obviate the need for a series of blocks in patients with vascular insufficiency or post herpetic neuralgia.[8]

SUCCESSFUL SYMPATHETIC BLOCK

A successful sympathetic block to the head and neck can be recognized by the Horner's syndrome, which includes Ptosis, Meiosis, Enophthalmos, and Anhidrosis. It may also cause conjunctival injection, nasal congestion.

However the presence of Horner's syndrom does not always indicate complete interruption of the sympathetic innervation of the upper extremity.

The following signs indicate effective sympathetic blockade of the upper extremity:
- Dilatation of veins in the upper extremity.
- Elevation of the temperature of the skin by 1 to 3° measured by Thermography or contact thermometry that is good except for the patients with elevated temperature.
- Increase in the skin resistance [Sympathogalvanic response].

Malmqvist et al[9] recommended that successful sympathetic block should satisfy five criteria, which include:
a. Horner's syndrome within 300 seconds.
b. Final skin temperature of 34°C or more, assuming an original temperature of 32° C or lower, i.e. 1 to 3° temperature increase.
c. An increase in blood flow by 50% or more from preblock status.
d. An increase in skin resistance by 13° or more from preblock on the ulnar and radial side of the blocked extremity.
e. Pulse amplitude changes, which are difficult to quantify.

Microneurography is a direct but invasive test requiring elaborate equipment and experience. Temperature measurement is the most widely used technique to assess complete sympathectomy of the affected side.

Selection of the Level of the Sympathetic Block

Matsumotos and Malmqvist et al reported that blockade at the level of C6 vertebra produced more successful sympathetic blockade to the head and neck with less success of sympathetic block of the upper extremity. C7 level block produces more successful block of the upper extremity. More appropriately, a sympathetic block by posterior approach to T2-T3 is more reliable for the upper extremity.

Any local anesthetic can be used but a smaller volume (1-2 ml) will help the operator to predict the response to radiofrequency ablation or chemical ablation. Precise injection using fluoroscopy or MRI guidance is therefore vital.

Post-procedure Care

The patient should be given a 15° head up position for about 10 to 15 minutes. Patients often have a lumpy feeling in the throat and should be kept nil by mouth for at least four hours. They also need to be reassured about the signs of Horner's syndrome which disappear by about 2 hours.

Complications

These can be classified into three categories as follows:

Technical Complications

- Vasovagal attacks
- Injury to the nerves and nearby viscera during insertion
- Injury to brachial plexus
- Trauma to the trachea or oesophagus [mediastinal or surgical emphysema]
- Injury to the pleura or lung [pneumo/hemothorax]
- Injury of the thoracic duct on the left side
- Bleeding or local hematoma: Airway compression
- Post procedure neuritis in 10 to 15% patients lasting 3 to 6 weeks.

Infectious Complications

- Cellulitis
- Osteitis
- Local abscess.

Pharmacological Complications

These can be related to the dose, volume and site of deposition of local anesthetic.

- Recurrent laryngeal nerve palsy: Hoarseness of voice, feeling of lump in throat
- Respiratory difficulty due to phrenic nerve palsy
- Somatic blockade of brachial plexus roots due to spillage
- Intraarterial injection into vertebral or carotid artery-seizures
- Injection into the intrathecal or epidural space
- Bradyarrhythmias and hypotension
- Cerebral air embolism.

    The most feared complications of the block are intraspinal injection or seizures triggered by intravascular injection. If these occur one has to institute resuscitative measures including intubation. Oxygen and mechanical ventilation are required till the local anesthetic wears off and patient resumes breathing. Mild sedation and reassurance may be needed to allay anxiety. I.V. fluids and vasopressors may be given, as required. The effects are generally self-limiting.

Chemical Neurolysis

The approach is similar to the stellate ganglion block performed at the level of C7. A 22 G needle is introduced at the C7 level at the junction of the transverse process with the vertebra. After confirming a good spread of the dye a total of 3 to 5 ml is injected. In AP view it should spread to inferior cervical ganglion cephalad, first thoracic sympathetic ganglion caudal.[6] In lateral view it should spread to retropharyngeal space in front of the longus colli muscle. A mixture of 2.5 ml of 6% phenol, 1 ml of 40 mg triamcinolone and 1.5% of 0.5% ropivacaine has been suggested. Head is maintained in elevated position for 30 minutes to prevent spread of phenol to the other structures.

Radiofrequency Neurolysis

This technique in experienced hands can provide long-term attenuation from pain in safer way, as it can be very precise having minimum effects on the adjacent vital structures.[10]

A 20 or 22 G special insulated blunt needle with 5 mm active tip is introduced through a special angiocatheter at the junction of the transverse process with the vertebral body. The depth and direction should be confirmed with AP and lateral views. Correct placement of the tip may be confirmed also by injecting a small amount of the contrast medium. A sensory (50 Hz, 0.9 V) and a motor (2Hz, 2V) stimulation trial must be performed. This helps in ruling out placement close to the phrenic nerve (lateral) and the recurrent laryngeal nerve (anterior and medial). While motor stimulation is performed, the patient should say "ee" to ensure preservation of the motor function. An 80° C lesion for 60 seconds is delivered. The needle is then redirected to the most medial aspect of the transverse process in the same plane. Motor and sensory stimulation is repeated to ensure safety. A third and final lesion should be directed at the upper portion of the junction of the transverse process and the body of C7.

Potential complications of radiofrequency lesioning are similar to those caused by stellate injection. Some specific ones are persistent Horner's syndrome, injury to the phrenic nerve, recurrent laryngeal nerve, neuritis (10-15% patients lasting 3-6 weeks) and vertebral artery injury.

Postsympathectomy Syndrome

Post sympathectomy neuralgia is a poorly understood painful condition, which occurs in up to 50% of patients undergoing sympathectomy. This is proposed to be a complex neuropathic and central deafferentation and reafferentation syndrome.[11] This can occur anywhere from few days to weeks following chemical or surgical sympathectomy. This is characterized by deep, aching pain with superficial burning and hyperesthesia, which may or may not respond to narcotic analgesics. Tricyclic antidepressants may help reduce the incidence of postsympathectomy neuralgia. Antiepileptic drugs like Phenytoin, Carbamazepine or Gabapentin may be useful to reduce spontaneous pain and allodynia. Mexiletine and I.V. lignocaine may help some patients. Occasionally invasive therapies like sympathetic block or more complete sympathectomy can also help.

CONCLUSION

Stellate ganglion block is one of the most frequently performed procedure in the practice of chronic pain. It can provide good diagnostic, therapeutic and prognostic value. It is strongly recommended to perform the block under fluoroscopic guidance. It can produce complete sympathectomy to the head and neck structures but only a partial sympathetic block of the upper extremity in some patients with variation in anatomy. Here T2-T3 sympathectomy may be desirable.

REFERENCES

1. Kappis M. Weitere erfahrungen mit der sympathectomie. Klin Wehr 1923;2:1441.
2. Brumm F. Die paravertebral injektion zur bekaempfung visceraler schmerzen. Wien Klin Aschsch 1924;37:511.
3. Warfield CA, Bajwa ZH. Principles and Practice of Pain Medicine, TATA McGraw Hill 2005;696-8.
4. Elias M. Review Article-Cervical Sympathetic and Stellate Ganglion Blocks. Pain Physician 2000;3:294-304.
5. Ellis H. Feldman S. Anatomy for the anaesthetists, (3rd edn). Oxford blackwell scientific publications 1979;256-62.
6. Hogan Q, Erickson S, Haddox D et al. The spread of solution during the stellate ganglion block. Regional anaesthesia 1992;17:78-83.
7. Elias M. The anterior approach for thoracic sympathetic ganglion block using a curved needle. Pain clinic 2000;12:17-24.
8. Elias M, Chakerian M. Repeated stellate ganglion block using a catheter for paediatric herpes zoster ophthalmicus. Anaesthesiology 1994; 1994:950-52.
9. Malmqvist El, Bengtsson M, Sorenson J. Efficacy of stellate ganglion block: A clinical study with bupivacaine. Reg Anaes 1992;17:340-47.
10. Geurts JW, Stolker RJ. Percutaneous radiofrequency lesion of the stellate ganglion in the treatment of pain in the upper extremity reflex sympathetic dystrophy. Pain clinic 1993;6:17-25.
11. Kramis RC, Roberts WJ, Gillette RG. Post-sympathectomy neuralgia: Hypotheses on peripheral and central neural mechanisms. Pain 1996;64;1-9.

Fifteen

Nerve Blocks for the Scalp and Injections

Tilottama Mangeshikar

SENSORY SUPPLY OF THE SCALP

Six Sensory Nerve Branches of Either the Trigeminal Nerve or the Cervical Nerve Supply to the Scalp

- The supratrochlear nerve is a branch of the ophthalmic division of the trigeminal nerve. This nerve supplies the scalp in the medial plane at the frontal region up to the vertex.
- The supraorbital nerve is also a branch of the ophthalmic division of the trigeminal nerve. This nerve supplies the scalp at the front, lateral to the supratrochlear nerve distribution, up to the vertex.
- The zygomaticotemporal nerve is a branch of the maxillary division of the trigeminal nerve and supplies the scalp over the temple region.
- The auriculotemporal nerve is a branch of the mandibular division of the trigeminal nerve and supplies the skin over the temporal region of the scalp.
- The lesser occipital nerve is a branch of the cervical plexus (C2), which supplies the scalp over the lateral occipital region.
- The greater occipital nerve is a branch of the posterior ramus of the second cervical nerve. This nerve supplies the scalp in the median plane at the occipital region up to the vertex.

Motor Supply

The frontal branch of the facial nerve supplies the frontal bellies of the occipitofrontalis muscle, and the auricular branch of the facial nerve supplies the occipital bellies of the muscle.

Blocks described:
- Deep cervical plexus block
- Superficial cervical plexus block
- Greater occipital nerve block
- Lesser occipital nerve block
- Great auricular nerve block
- Botulinum toxin A injections for migraine.

Deep Cervical Plexus Block (Figs 15.1 and 15.2)

The transverse processes of C2 to C4 are located 0.5 to 1 cm posterior to the line joining the mastoid process with Chassaignac's tubercle. The first needle is placed at C4 as this is the easiest landmark to identify and serves to guide placement of the C3 and C2 needles. The index finger of the free hand is used to palpate the transverse process of C4 and compress the soft tissues. Firm pressure may be required to feel the transverse processes. The palpating index finger is then fixed in place on the transverse process while a 1 ½" to 2" blunt 22-gauge regional needle is placed just off the tip of the index finger at C4 in a caudal, medial, and slightly posterior direction. A distinct bony endpoint is felt as the needle encounters the transverse process of C4. This usually occurs at about 1" to 1¼" in a normal sized adult. The depth required to reach the transverse processes of C3 and C2 increases, respectively.

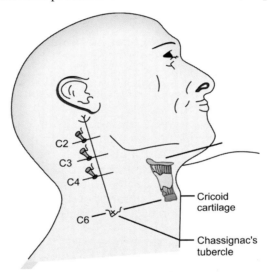

Fig. 15.1: Deep cervical plexus: surface marking

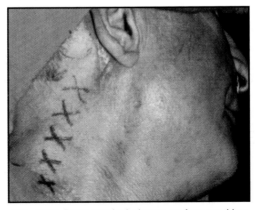

Fig. 15.2: Deep cervical plexus: surface marking
needles entry position

Having placed the C4 needle, needles are now placed in a similar fashion at C3 and C2. The C4 and C3 needles' direction and depth are used to guide placement of the C3 and C2 needles, respectively. If the patient has a large neck, a 2" blunt 22 gauge needle will likely be required to reach the transverse process of C2. An attempt is made to place all three needles correctly before any local anesthetic agent is given. If blood appears in the hub of a needle, the needle should be replaced prior to injection of local anesthetic. If needle placement is difficult, a single needle at one level (preferably located at C3), has been used successfully. The total volume of local anesthetic (15 to 24 ml) that would be injected with three needles, is now injected at the single needle location. Paresthesias may be elicited but are not needed or sought to perform the block.

With the three needles successfully placed, the C2 needle is connected (Fig. 15.3) to the control syringe containing the local anesthetic. With the syringe attached, the needle is again confirmed to be resting upon the transverse process. The syringe-needle unit is then carefully withdrawn by 1 to 2 mm. With needle stabilization, and following a negative aspiration test for blood (vertebral artery) and CSF, 5 to 8 ml of the local anesthetic solution is injected. The C2 needle is removed and the control syringe is reloaded with the same amount of local anesthetic. The procedure is repeated for the C3 and C4 needles, respectively. The C2 needle is injected first, as it's placement is the most difficult of the three needles, and repositioning the C2 needle would be difficult after the C3 and C4 needles have been injected and their needles removed.

Alternatively, the clinician may opt to use block needles with attached extension tubing. This eliminates the need to grasp and stabilize the needle for attachment to the syringe, and minimizes the chance of dislodging a neighboring needle by the operator's finger.

Complications of a deep cervical plexus block include possible intraarterial injection of local anesthetic into the vertebral artery resulting in an immediate loss of consciousness, seizure, or temporary blindness.

A caudad needle direction is essential to minimize the risk of an inadvertent epidural or intrathecal injection of local anesthetic.

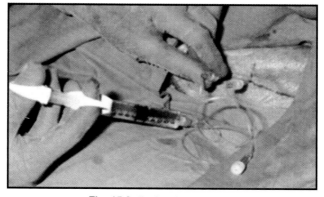

Fig. 15.3: Performing the block

The phrenic nerve may also be anesthetized when performing the deep cervical plexus block resulting in a temporary paralysis of the ipsilateral diaphragm. Usually this is of no clinical significance.

The cervical fascia separates the cervical sympathetic chain and the recurrent laryngeal nerve from the deep cervical plexus. If local anesthetic is injected more superficially a temporary recurrent laryngeal nerve palsy (hoarseness) and/or Horner's syndrome (ptosis, miosis, anhydrosis) may be observed on the same side.

If local anesthetic is injected into the brachial plexus sheath, a brachial plexus block may be produced.

SUPERFICIAL CERVICAL PLEXUS BLOCK

The external jugular vein crosses the posterior border of the SCM muscle belly at it's midpoint (approximately at the C4 level). A 25 gauge spinal needle is inserted perpendicular to the skin at the junction of the lateral border of the SCM muscle and the external jugular vein. The tip of the spinal needle is advanced to a depth equal to the thickness of the SCM muscle belly. At this depth, the superficial cervical plexus is emerging from the neck. Four ml of local anesthetic solution is injected at this point.

The spinal needle is then angulated to allow cephalad and caudad subcutaneous tunnelling along the lateral border of the clavicular head of the SCM muscle. Approximately 3 to 4 ml of local anesthetic is injected in each direction. Care is taken to avoid puncture, and inadvertent injection of local anesthetic into the external jugular vein.

GREATER AND LESSER OCCIPITAL NERVE BLOCKS

Anatomy (Fig. 15.4)

The **greater occipital nerve** arises from the dorsal primary ramus of the second and third cervical nerve. It gives sensation to the medial portion of the posterior scalp. The *lesser occipital nerve* arises from the ventral primary rami of the second and third cervical roots and give supply to the cranial surface of the pinna and adjacent scalp.

It arises from the second cervical nerve, sometimes also from the third; it curves around and ascends along the posterior border of the sternocleidomastoid.

Near the cranium it perforates the deep fascia, and is continues upward along the side of the head behind the ear, supplying the skin and communicating with the greater occipital, the great auricular, and the posterior auricular branch of the facial.

The lesser occipital varies in size, and is sometimes duplicated.

It gives off an auricular branch, which supplies the skin of the upper and back part of the auricula, communicating with the mastoid branch of the great auricular.

This branch is occasionally derived from the *greater occipital nerve*. Disorder in this nerve causes *occipital neuralgia*.

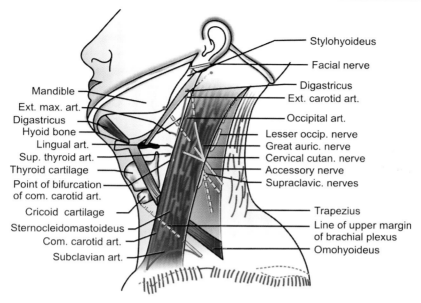

Fig. 15.4: Anatomy of occipital nerve and its branches

Technique (Fig. 15.5)

The greater occipital nerve runs with the occipital artery. The nerve is identified at its point of entry to the scalp, along the superior nuchal line midway between the mastoid process and the occipital protuberance. The patient will report pain upon compression: the point at which maximal tenderness is elicited can be used as the injection site. The scalp is cleansed with an alcohol swab; 6 mg betamethasone (1 ml) is drawn into a syringe containing 1 ml 2% lidocaine. A 25-gauge 5/8 inch needle is used for the block. The needle is directed toward the occiput until bony resistance is felt, thus ensuring that the subarachnoid space is not entered. About 0.6 ml

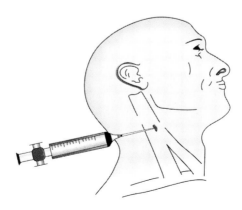

Fig. 15.5: Entry point for greater occipital nerve

is injected; the type of the needle is then withdrawn to just under the skin and redirected about 5 degrees laterally and then again medially, to deposit about 0.6 ml into each site to ensure a successful block. On completion of the injection, the injected area is massaged and compressed to spread the steroid suspension so that at least some of it bathes the nerve trunk. Hypesthesia should appear within 1 to 2 minutes, extending forward on the scalp to the interaural line. The lesser occipital nerve can be blocked by injecting 1 inch inferior and medial to this area. The occipital artery can often be palpated and used as a landmark for injection of both areas.

GREATER AURICULAR NERVE BLOCK

Anatomy

The greater auricular nerve arises from the ventral rami of C2 and C3. It passes Erb's point to supply the skin in the region of the ear, angle of the jaw, and over the parotid gland.

Technique (Fig. 15.6)

The material for performing this block is standard neurostimulation needle, with court bevel of 50 mm (24G) connected to a syringe of Luer Lock. A cutaneous pen marker.

For the puncture the patient must be positioned with the head turned towards the opposite side. The first reference mark is the mastoid (M in Fig. 15.6), to mark it with the pen; the second reference mark P – Fig. 15.6, the lateral edge of SCM on the cricoid level. The block will be done on the line joining these 2 points. The puncture point is done to 10 mm above the point of SCM; the needle passes in and moves towards the mastoid, injecting throughout. The injection is very slow with 7 ml of anesthetic solution, while advancing towards the mastoid. A discrete massage supports the diffusion of the product.

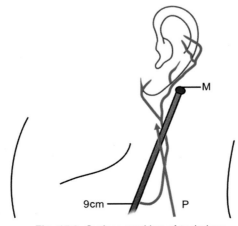

Fig. 15.6: Surface marking of technique

The territory supplied by the great auricular nerve is external ear, in its inferior and posterior zone (half inferior external ear), as well as a small cutaneous territory of the angle of the mandible. No complication is noted, except, if the puncture is too deep, a diffusion on the facial nerve is possible, with a transitory paresis.

BOTULINUM TOXIN A INJECTIONS FOR MIGRAINE

Botulinum toxin is a neurotoxin produced by clostridium botulinum, the bacteria that thrive in poorly sterilized canned food and produce the severe food poisoning called botulism. These are the toxin that paralyze nerves by blocking the release of a substance called acetylcholine - which blocks the muscles and prevents them from contracting thereby causing paralysis. The substance which is ingested in spoiled food and causes the illness is known as botulism.

However, in therapeutic uses, Botox is injected directly into the muscle rather than absorbed into the bloodstream. The dose is a fraction of those which cause botulism.

Botox is well known for its use in treatment of wrinkles. It has approval for use in treating facial tics and spasms, dystonia and other forms of spasticity in cerebral palsy for example, its tolerability and safety record for these uses are excellent. The principle behind its use in this case is to relax tense or spastic muscles by blocking acetylcholine release which stimulates muscle contraction.

The discovery of Botox for treatment of migraine was quite by accident. Several patients who were using Botox for injection of wrinkles also happened to have migraine. They reported improvement in their headaches following injection of Botox to their brow and forehead muscles.

The mechanism of action is not entirely clear. One possibility is that Botox may decrease muscle contraction that may act as a trigger to migraine. Another theory is that Botox may act on a brain related chemical like substance P which is involved in pain and migraine mechanisms.

Careful trials studying migraine and chronic headache patients continue to examine the efficacy of Botox. Several small trials have been completed and results of a large placebo controlled trial are pending.

The average dose is 100-200 units. The onset of action is usually within the first 2 to 3 weeks of injection however patients may require a set of 2 to 3 injections before maximum benefit is seen. Injections are spaced at 12 week intervals.

Safety is always a concern. However, Botox' record since 1989 is excellent. There is no systemic absorption as there is with oral medication, therefore no systemic side effects are seen. Drooping eyelids can occur with improper injection technique but are transient.

Some Published Uses of Botulinum Toxin Type A

- Achalasia
- Blepharospasm

- Cervical dystonia
- Essential tremor.

Headache and Migraine

- Hemifacial spasm
- Hyperhydrosis
- Myofascial pain.

Occupational Dystonia

Pain (muscle spasm)

- Spasmodic dystonia
- Strabismus
- Spasticity
- Cerebral palsy
- Multiple sclerosis
- Stroke
- Traumatic brain injury
- Wrinkles.

Technique and Sites (Figs 15.7 to 15.9)

- 2 CC saline for dilution
- 20 G 2" needle to draw up toxin
- Change needle
- 30 G ½ inch needle
- Skin prep with isopropyl alcohol
- Swab stick for minor bleeding
- Finger pressure on all injections sites.

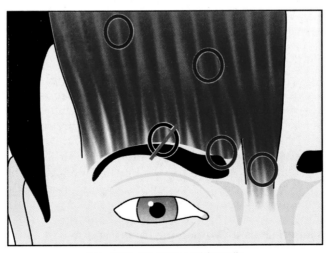

Fig. 15.7: Procerus and frontalis

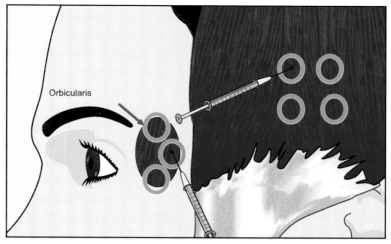

Fig. 15.8: Temporalis and orbicularis

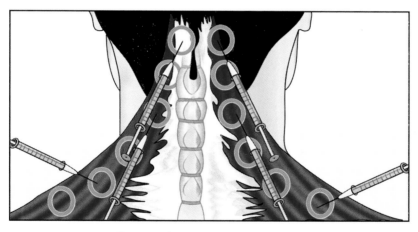

Fig. 15.9: Occipitalis and neck muscles

Section D

Chest and Thorax

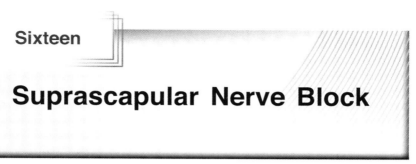

Sixteen

Suprascapular Nerve Block

Jitendra Jain

INTRODUCTION

Shoulder pain is common in the community, affecting 15 to 30% of adults at any one time. Shoulder pain causes include degenerative disease affecting the glenohumeral and acromioclavicular joints and supporting soft tissue structures. Also in the list are inflammatory diseases such as rheumatoid arthritis (RA), seronegative spondyloarthropathies, and crystal arthropathies. Because of pain, a progressive loss of movement resulting in a loss of function. These are the patients for which commonly suprascapular nerve block was done. Also patient of shoulder reconstruction and replacement are also benefiting from the suprascapular nerve block for early range of motion and rehabilitation.

ANATOMY

Nerve fibers of suprascapular nerve originates from C5 , C6 and sometimes also contributed by C4. Nerve leaves brachial plexus, passing inferiorly and posterior under the coracoclavicular ligament through the suprascapular notch.

Blood vessels accompany the suprascapular nerve in the suprascapular notch. It provides muscular insertion to supraspinatus and infraspinatus of the rotator cuff and sensory innervation of the shoulder joint and AC joint. (Figs 16.1 and 16.2).

Indications

- Adhesive capsulitis
- Frozen shoulder[1]
- Acute shoulder pain
- Cancer pain and palliation
- Post shoulder reconstruction/replacement
- Rehabilitation of chronic arm or hand problem patients for shoulder movement.

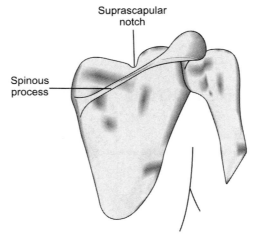

Fig. 16.1: Diagrammatic posterior view representing suprascapular notch where the suprascapular nerve lies

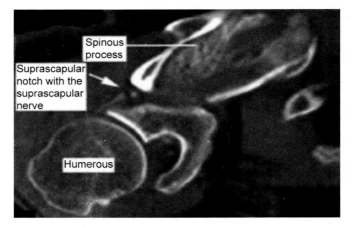

Fig. 16.2: CT scan showing suprascapular notch with the white round suprascapular nerve in it

Contraindication

- Coagulopathies
- Local infection.

Equipment and Drugs

- 2 ml, 5 ml and 10 ml syringes
- 18 G, 24 G needles for aspiration and skin infiltration respectively
- 10 cm radiofrequency (RF) needle with 10 mm active tip preferably blunt

- Local anesthetic lignocaine and bupivacaine[2]
- Triamcinolone or methylprednisolone, i.e. depot steroids[3]
- Phenol
- Pain management radiofrequency generator [4,5]
- C-arm (Fluoroscopy).

Preparation

Diagnostic shoulder examination and needle entry points should be examined before hand. Diagnostic blood investigation depending on the patient could be asked for.

Usually this procedure is done under local anesthesia and if RF is planned then conscious sedation could be used. For that ASA guidelines could be followed.

Procedure

Patient is in the prone position. C-arm is used to locate the suprascapular notch. Usually the trajectory is lateral to midline and cephalocaudal to have a good view of the suprascapular notch (Fig. 16.3). Once after getting a good vision of suprascapular notch 1½ inch needle or RF needle is used in gun barrel vision just below the notch after infiltrating skin with lignocaine. Once it hits the bone just below the notch needle is guided to walk of the scapular body to enter the notch (Fig. 16.4). Usually within 4 to 5 cm one should be able make contact with the body of the scapula. Paresthesia might be encountered around shoulder region. If there is no paresthesia or if the stimulator facility is available then stimulating suprascapular nerve is a good idea. One should not go more than 1/2 inch after walking off the scapular body into the notch. You might be puncturing the pleura. Iohexol is used to confirm the position of the needle and also to check if there is no intravascular spread if one is planning neurolysis. Using nerve stimulator for local block injection or phenol is a good idea to reconfirm the position of the needle.

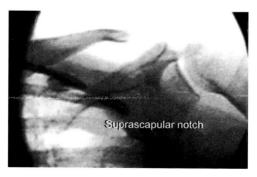

Fig. 16.3: Showing C-arm picture of suprascapular notch. Needle needs to be directed to the notch in Gun barrel view

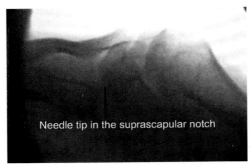

Needle tip in the suprascapular notch

Fig. 16.4: Needle in the suprascapular notch, needs to be confirmed with contrast and stimulatory parameters so as confirm the needle proximity to the suprascapular nerve

Local Anesthetic Block

10 ml of 0.25 to 0.5% bupivacaine with depot steroid 40 to 80 mg.

Neurolysis

4 to 5 ml of 6% phenol after confirming with local block.

Radiofrequency

Sensory stimulation at 0.3 to 0.6 V of 50Hz and motor stimulations double of sensory parameters at 2Hz is done to confirm the placement. Once confirmed pulsed radiofrequency at 42°C for 120 sec and 2 such cycles is used.

Post-procedure taking the benefit of pain relief cautious physiotherapy and rehabilitation program is advisable for almost all patients unless contraindicated.

Complication and Caution

* Intravascular injections and local anesthetic toxicity
* Pneumothorax
* Suprascapular nerve damage
* Caution to post block shoulder weakness and decreased sensation.

It is simple block and has a very good utility for shoulder pain due to degenerative problems, trauma, cancer or surgery.

REFERENCES

1. Shaffer B, Tibone JE, Kerlan RK. Frozen shoulder: A long-term follow-up. J Bone Joint Surg 1992;74A:738-46.
2. Gado K, Emery P. Modified suprascapular nerve block with bupivacaine alone effectively controls chronic shoulder pain in patients with rheumatoid arthritis. Ann Rheum Dis 1993;52:215-8.
3. Van der Heijden GJ, van der Windt DA, Kleijnen J, et al. Steroid injections for shoulder disorders: A systemic review of randomized clinical trials. Br J Gen Pract 1996;46:309-16.

4. Rohof OJJM, Dongen VCPCV. Pulsed radiofrequency of the suprascapular nerve in the treatment of chronic intractable shoulder pain in 2nd world congress of pain. Istanbul: Blackwell Science: 2001.

5. Rinoo V Shah, Gabor B Racz. A Case Report. 2003;6;503-6. Pulsed mode radiofrequency lesioning of the suprascapular nerve for the treatment of chronic shoulder pain: Pain physician journal.

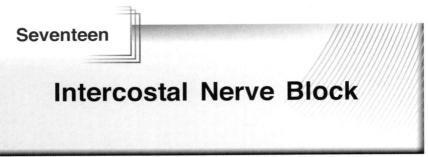

Seventeen

Intercostal Nerve Block

Jitendra Jain

INTRODUCTION

It is a very important tool to manage the patients with pain originating from chest wall and upper abdomen. There are various medical conditions for which this block could be considered.

ANATOMY

The intercostal nerves are composed of the anterior branch of the first till the twelfth thoracic nerve.[1] The typical ones are from 3rd till 11th thoracic nerve. Slight variations in the typical course are seen with first, 2nd and twelfth intercostal nerve.

The typical one (Fig. 17.1) gives four well defined branches in its way starting from the thoracic root till the intercostal nerve. First is branches to and fro from the thoracic sympathetic chain, i.e. Grey rami communicans. Second branch is the posterior cutaneous branch which supplies the paravertebral skin and muscles. Third is lateral cutaneous nerve arising just anterior to the midaxillary line. This branch subcutaneous fiber might overlap with the posterior and anterior cutaneous branches. Final branch is the anterior cutaneous branch which actually gives cutaneous innervation to the midline of the chest and abdomen.

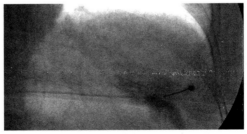

Fig. 17.1: Showing a typical intercostal nerve giving various branches along its course after exiting the dorsal foramen

Twelfth intercostal nerve is called subcostal nerve which runs along abdominal wall and joins L1 to finally continue as iliohypogastric and ilioinguinal nerves.

T1 contributes to brachial plexus while T2 and T3 sends cutaneous branches to medial aspect of arm as intercostobrachial nerve.

Indications

- Fractured ribs
- Sternotomy[2]
- Thoracotomy[3]
- Post herpetic neuralgia
- Post surgical thoracic or abdominal nerve entrapment
- Upper abdominal surgeries
- Appendectomy.

Contraindication

- Local infection
- Coagulopathy.

Equipment and Drugs

- 25G ¾ inch needle
- 22G 1½ inch needle
- 5 cm RF needle with 5 mm active tip
- 2 ml, 3 ml and 5 ml syringe
- 1 to 2% lignocaine
- 0.25%-0.5% bupivacaine
- Depot steroids
- 6% phenol
- Absolute alcohol
- Radiofrequency generator.

Preparation

Preprocedure history and physical examination of the local area before intercostal block is a must. It mainly to understand to level at which block is to be given and if at all there are any anatomical changes because of pathology or surgery.

Coagulation profile and requisite preoperative blood investigation of the patient could be done depending on the patient.

For this block usually sedation is not needed unless a patient is restless or radiofrequency is planned.

Position

- Lateral
- Prone
- Sitting.

The rib to be blocked is identified and local anesthesia with lignocaine is given along posterior axillary line or fluoroscopy is used after preparing the skin with antiseptic. Inferior border of the rib is identified and if doing blind rib is hit with the needle or fluoroscopy is used for guidance. After hitting the bone needle is withdrawn till subcutaneous level and guided till the inferior bony contact is lost. As soon as the bony contact is lost needle is advance for about 1to 3 mm not more otherwise pleura might be punctured. Placement is confirmed by stimulating and also by injecting dye at that level (Figs 17.2 and 17.3). Once confirmed then desired treatment modality is delivered.

Drugs Injected

- 0.5 to 1ml of 6% phenol or absolute alcohol.
- 1 to 2 ml of 0.25 to 0.5% bupivacaine with or without depot steroid 40 mg.
- Radiofrequency ablation, pulsed is preferred or lower temperature heating with RF is preferred. Cryoablation[4] can also be done if facility is available (Fig. 17.3).
- Continuous block for post operative patients can be done by placing catheter.

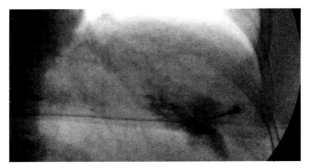

Fig. 17.2: Showing needle placement in the subcostal groove with contrast spread in the area

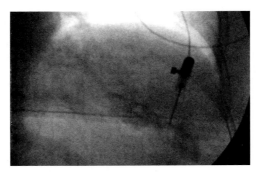

Fig. 17.3: Fluoroscopic picture showing needle placement in the subcostal groove in proximity to the intercostal nerve and undergoing radiofrequency ablation

Complications

- Pneumothorax
- Local anesthetic allergy or toxicity due to proximity to blood vessels
- Infection.

Alcohol block if possible can be avoided as it might cause post procedure neuritis.

REFERENCES

1. Moore DC. Anatomy of the intercostal nerve: Its importance during thoracic surgery. Am J Surg 1982;144:371-3.
2. Perttunen K, Tasmuth T, Kalso E. Chronic pain after thoracic surgery: A follow-up study. Acta Anaesthesiol Scand 1999;43:563-7.
3. Katz J, Jackson M, Kavanagh BP, Sandler AN. Acute pain after thoracic surgery predicts long-term post-thoracotomy pain. Clin J Pain 1996;12:50-55.
4. Pastor J, Morales P, Cases E, Cordero P, Piqueras A, Galan G, Paris F. Evaluation of intercostal cryoanalgesia versus conventional analgesia in postthoracotomy pain. Respiration 1996;63:241-5.

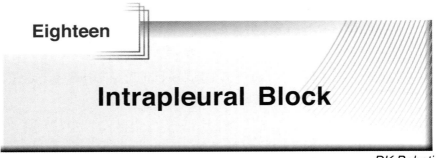

Eighteen

Intrapleural Block

INTRODUCTION

The lung is covered with two layers of pleura. One is parietal and second is pleural. The friction of both the layers while breathing causes pain. This often leads to a peculiar situation for a patient, i.e. if he breathes heavily then intensity of pain increases due to friction of both the pleura and if he hold the breath due to fear of pain then chances of CO_2 retention and even hypoxia are there. Pleura are supplied by all the intercostals nerves. There is retrograde diffusion of local anesthetic back towards intercostal nerves.

Indications

- Carcinoma of lung
- Carcinoma of gall bladder
- Secondary in the lung
- Post herpetic neuralgia
- Post surgical thoracic or abdominal nerve entrapment
- Upper abdominal surgeries
- Post thoracotomy pain.[1]

Contraindications

- Patient unable, unwilling to consent or uncooperative patient
- Known allergy to contrast
- Local or systemic infection
- Coagulopathy
- Pregnancy
- Concurrent use of anticoagulants
- Coexisting disease producing significant CVS or respiratory compromise
- Immunosuppression.

Equipment/Types and Sizes of Needle

- C-arm fluoroscopy or CT scan along with monitoring and resuscitation facility.
- 26-gauge for skin infiltration and deep infiltration of local anesthetic.
- Epidural set (16-guage needle with epidural catheter and filter).

Drugs and Concentration

- Inj. lignocaine- 2% - (xylocard- preservative free)
- Inj. iohexol (omnipaque), a water soluble contrast
- Inj. bupivacaine 0.25%
- Inj. phenol in glycerine- 6 to 10% or Inj. tetracycline for pleurodesis.

Pre-operative Preparation

Informed consent.
Investigations complete blood count, bleeding time and clotting time.
Secure an intravenous line.
Monitoring of BP, SaO_2, and ECG .
An antibiotic cover.

Procedure

Step 1   Patient in sitting position with arm rested on mayo's trolley or lateral decubitus position. After preparing the site, identify 7, 8, 9th intercostal space and do the surfacing marking of 9th and 10th intercostal spaces (Figs 18.1 and 18.2).

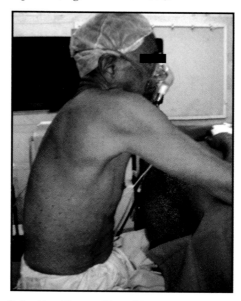

Fig. 18.1: Patient in sitting position with hand resting on Mayo's trolly

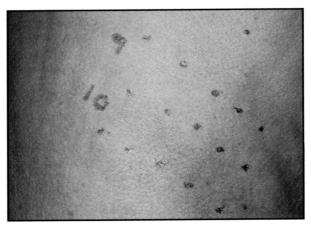

Fig. 18.2: Surface marking of 9th and 10th intercostal space

In the 9th intercostal space at mid/post axillary line, under local anesthesia advance 16-gauge Tuohy needle and contact the rib.

Then walk of superiorly about 3 to 5 mm with loss of resistance technique using normal saline or put a drop of saline at hub of needle (Hanging drop) to demonstrate the movement of saline drop with respiration.

Step 2 Confirm the needle position under fluoroscopy anteriolateral view. After repeated negative aspiration inject water soluble dye Inj. omnipaque 3 to 5 cc. Confirm the spread of the dye under fluoroscopy. Inject 3 to 4 cc of Inj. xyloacaine preservative free 3 to 5 cc.

Step 3 Now slowly introduce epidural catheter through epidural needle about 3 to 5 cm into the pleura. Once again inject about 2 cc Inj. omnipaque into the epidural catheter and confirm the spread of dye under fluoroscopy in both anterior posterior and lateral view (Figs 18.3 to 18.5).

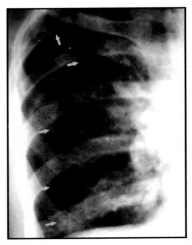

Fig. 18.3: Catheter (as shown by the arrows) in pleural space

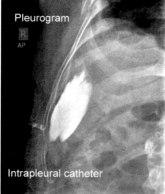

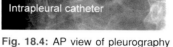

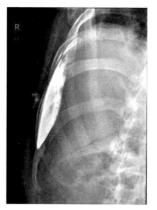

Fig. 18.4: AP view of pleurography   **Fig. 18.5:** Lateral view of pleurography

Step 4   Tunnel the catheter into the adjacent skin. Fix it with adhesive tape (Fig. 18.6).

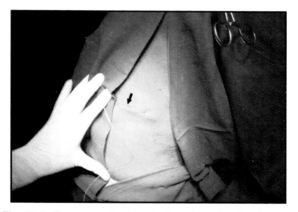

Fig. 18.6: Tunneling of epidural catheter in intrapleural space

Step 5   Inject the Inj. tetracycline 8 to 10 cc through epidural catheter slowly. Flush epidural catheter with Inj. bupivacaine 0.25% 4 to 5 cc.

Step 6   Shift to recovery area and monitor the vital parameters for 2 to 3 hours.

COMPLICATIONS

- Pneumothorax
- Local anesthetic allergy or toxicity due to proximity to blood vessels
- Infection.

REFERENCE

1. Bachman-Mennenga B, Biscoping J, Kuhn DEM, et al. Intercostal, interpleural analgesia, thoracic epidural block or systemic opioid application for pain relief after thoracotomy? Eur J Cardiothorac Surg 1993;7:12-8.

Section E

Abdomen and Pelvis

Nineteen

Celiac Plexus Block

DK Baheti

INTRODUCTION

Kappis[1] in 1914 first described the percutaneous posterior approach for the block of splanchnic nerves and celiac plexus for surgical anesthesia. He in 1918 reported series of 200 cases with the same approach.

Jones[2] in 1957 used alcohol neurolysis for long lasting relief of abdominal pain. Bride Baugh, et al[3] reported the role of neurolytic celiac plexus block for abdominal malignancy.

The posterior approach is still widely used approach for the block of celiac plexus and splanchnic nerves.

Abdominal pain is one of the most common symptoms by contrast to other areas of the body, as abdominal organs have poorly developed sensory systems and that is the problem for patient to describe the pain and for physician to localize the pain. The purpose of the pain is to protect the organ and patient form injury.

Abdominal viscera are relatively insensitive to many stimuli compared with a more sensitive organ such as the epidermis. In addition to the relative paucity of sensory nerve endings, as the same group of nerves may supply several viscera. There are very few well known nociceptive triggers in the abdominal cavity. These include abnormal distention or contraction of hollow organ walls, ischemia of visceral musculature, direct action of chemical substance on the mucosa, formation of allogenic mediators and traction or compression of ligaments, vessels or mesentery.

The visceral pain is transmitted from nociceptors found on the walls of the abdominal viscera via sympathetic and parasympathetic pathway. This pain is nonspecific because of wide divergence and relatively small number of afferent fibers innervating a large area with extensive ramification.

Patients usually have difficulty in localizing the source of pain and will describe as aching, cramping or burning that fluctuates in the intensity. Visceral pain is usually paroxysmal, colicky, deep, squeezing, and diffuse. The pain originating from visceral structures and innervated by celiac plexus can be effectively alleviated by blocking of celiac plexus. These structures are pancreas, liver, gallbladder, omentum, mesentery, and alimentary tract from stomach to the transverse portion of large colon.

An additional benefit to these patients may be effect of the celiac plexus block is on the gastric motility.

Indications

1. Any pain originating from upper abdominal viscera such as stomach, liver, gall bladder, kidney, spleen, pancreas, aortic lymphadenopathy, omental mass, retroperitoneal tumors.
2. Pain due to chronic pancreatitis, alcoholic pancreatitis.
3. Any chronic upper abdominal pain of unknown origin.

Contraindications

1. Receiving anticoagulation therapy or suffering from congenital abnormalities of coagulopathy.
2. Antiblastic cancer therapy.
3. Liver abnormalities associated with ethanol abuse.
4. The local skin infection at needle entry point or intra abdominal infection and sepsis, intestinal obstruction.
5. The use of alcohol as neurolytic agent should be avoided in patient with disulfiram therapy for alcohol abuse.

Equipment/Types and Sizes of Needle (Fig. 19.1)

- Procedure room with C-arm fluoroscopy or CT scan along with monitoring and resuscitation facility
- Radiofrequency lesion generator
- 26-gauge needle for skin infiltration and deep infiltration of local anesthetic
- 18-guage needle or 11 no. surgical blade for skin puncture to facilitate the insertion of blunt tip needle
- 20-guage 6″ long blunt tip needle or 22-gauge 6″ long needle.

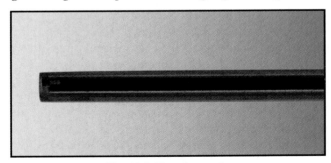

Fig. 19.1: Blunt tip needle

DRUGS AND CONCENTRATION

- Inj. lignocaine- 2%- (xylocard- preservative free)
- Absolute alcohol

- Normal saline
- Inj. bupivacaine 0.25%.

Procedure

Pre Operative Preparation

Any interventional procedures should be done with informed consent. These procedures are preferably done in procedure room or in operation theater. The investigations such as complete blood count, bleeding time and clotting time are necessary. An intravenous line is secured. The monitoring of BP, SaO_2, and ECG is mandatory. An antibiotic cover is necessary. The guidance of fluoroscopy, ultrasound, CT scan is useful.

There are many approaches to perform the celiac plexus block such as retrocrural, transcrural (uni or bilateral), transdiscal, transaortic, anterior approach, splanchnic denervation. It is the choice of pain specialist which approach he is comfortable with.

The author prefers posterior approach so it is given in detail step wise.

POSTERIOR APPROACH – COMMON AND PREFERRED APPROACH

Position and Landmarks (Fig. 19.2)

Step 1   In this approach the patient is in prone position with a pillow under the abdomen to reverse to thoracolumbar lordosis also this position increases the distance between costal margin and ileac crests and transverse processes of adjacent vertebral bodies.

The preloading of the patient with Inj. ringer lactate 500 to 1000 ml at the start of the procedure how ever it depend on pre operative hemodynamic status of the patient.

Step 2   The standard landmarks are ileac crests, 12th rib, and spinous process of T12 and L1 vertebrae. Moore recommended that intersection of 12th rib and lateral border of paraspinal muscles on both sides and spine of L1 vertebra which forms an isosceles triangle.

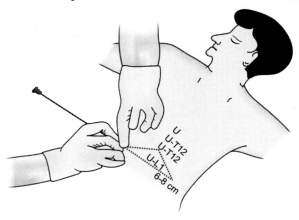

Fig. 19.2: Landmarks and needle entry

Step 3 The point of needle entry is either four finger breadth or 6 to 8 cm from midline. Inj. 2% lidocaine about 10 cc intradermally and deep into the various layers in the direction of the needle. Then in case of blunt needle make a skin niche with 18-gauge hypodermic needle or with 11 no. surgical blade to facilitate the entry of blunt needle.

Step 4 A 15 cm 20-gauge styleted short bevel or blunt tip needle are directed one side with 45 degree angle towards midline and cephalad to contact body of L1 vertebra. Then second needle on other side also inserted in the same manner as before. The position of the needle should be confirmed antero-posterior (Fig. 19.3) and lateral view (Fig. 19.4) under fluoroscopy or under CT scan.

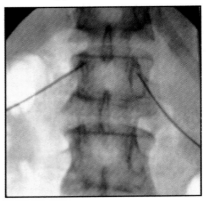

Fig. 19.3: Position of needles in AP view

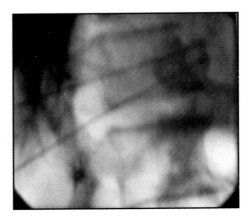

Fig. 19.4: Position of needles in lateral view

Step 5 In lateral view after repeated negative aspiration, one needle at a time should be redirected towards anterior border of L1 vertebra. The tip of the both needle should be about 1 to 2 cm ahead of anterior border of L1 vertebra. It is advised the tip of right side needle should be little ahead of the left as more fibers of the celiac plexus are on the right side.

Step 6 After repeated negative aspiration the 5 cc of 2% lidocaine injected to have immediate pain relief. At this stage there can be sudden fall of blood pressure, which can be treated either with Inj. mephenteramine sulphate 3 to 6 mgm or inj. Ringer Lactate 500 to 1000 cc.

Step 7 After repeated negative aspiration 5 cc radiopaque dye iohexol injected on each side and spread of the dye is confirmed under fluoroscopy or CT scan. The spread of the dye should restrict to the body of T12 and L1 vertebra (Figs 19.5 and 19.6). Both the pictures should be saved for documentation.

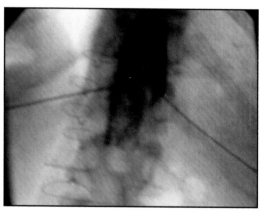

Fig. 19.5: Spread of dye AP view

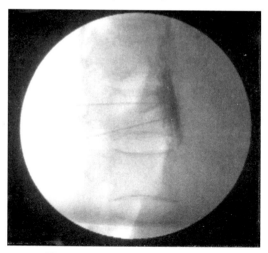

Fig. 19.6: Spread of dye lateral view

S Jain[4] suggested that if CT guidance is used, the contrast material should appear lateral to and behind the aorta. If contrast material is confined entirely to the retrocrural space, the needles should be advanced to the retrocrural space to minimize the risk of posterior spread of local anesthetic or neurolytic agent to the somatic nerve roots.

Step 8 Once again after repeated negative aspiration, a mixture of Inj. alcohol 50% with the Inj. bupivacaine 0.25%, 20 to 25 cc should be injected slowly on both sides. The needle should be withdrawn with stylet in order to avoid spillage of neurolytic agent in the track of the needle.

Step 9 The vital signs of the patient should be observed in the recovery for about 1 to 2 hours.

ANTERIOR APPROACH

This is done either under ultrasonographic or CT guidance. The needle entry is 1.5 cm below and 1.5 cm left of the xiphoid process. A 22 gauge 15 cm needle is directed perpendicular to the skin and advanced to the anterior to the aorta under ultrasonographic or CT guidance. If CT is used 3 to 4 cc of Inj. iohexol is used to confirm the spread of the dye and under ultrasonographic guidance 10 to 15 cc of saline is used confirm needle position. Then repeated negative 10 to 15 cc of 1% Inj. lidocaine is used to confirm the diagnostic block. Then after repeated negative aspiration 1 to 15 cc of absolute alcohol is injected. The needle is withdrawn with stylet.

INTRADISCAL APPROACH

The position of the patient is prone with a pillow under the abdomen and is to be done under fluoroscopy. The T12 - L1 level is identified. A single 15 cm 20-gauge styleted needle at a time is passed through the midline on either side.

The position of the needle anterior to the vertebral body is confirmed under fluoroscopy. The dye iohexol 5 cc is injected and spread of the dye is confirmed under fluoroscopy.

After repeated negative aspiration, a mixture of Inj. alcohol 50% with the Inj. bupivacaine 0.25%, 20 to 25 cc should be injected slowly on both sides.

The needle should be withdrawn with stylet in order to avoid spillage of neurolytic agent into the track of the needle.

COMPLICATIONS OF NEUROLYTIC CELIAC PLEXUS BLOCK

The iatrogenic complication reported during celiac plexus blocks are pneumothorax (two cases) by Brown[5]; partial lower extremity paralysis (One case) by Thomson et al.[6]; temporary paraplegia (One case) by Baheti.[7] Iatrogenic complications such as chylothorax, pleural effusion, renal injury and injury to veins also have been reported.

While performing lumbar sympathectomy Boas[8] reported 6% incidence of genitofemoral neuralgia, Cousins and associates[9] reported 35 patients with mild or severe neuralgia.

The neurological complications include disestesias, paresis in lower extremities, paraplegia due to ischemia, spinal neurolytic injection, spasm of anterior spinal artery.

The complications include abdominal pain, diarrhea, hypotension, pneumothorax, injury to vessels.

Other complications such as backache, intravascular or subarachnoid injection, neuralgia, muscle spasm are mentioned by P Raj et al.[10]

The role of sharp needle in above complications can not be ruled out.

The probable cause of above mentioned iatrogenic complications can be the use of a 6 inches or a 15 cm long needles (sharp tip or short bevel), which may results in a iatrogenic puncture of an internal organ like vein, pleura, peritoneum and etc. and as mentioned above, these iatrogenic complications have been reported in the literature from time to time.

EVOLUTION IN THE TECHNIQUE OF CPB

Since 1914 many advances have done in the performing of celiac plexus block such as various routes like anterior, transaortic, thoracoscopic, laparoscopic.

At the same time use of fluoroscopy, CT scan, ultrasound have made difference and celiac plexus block can be performed with more accuracy and long lasting pain relief can be produced. The use of non ionic dye has become useful guideline to confirm the spread of dye and chances of dye reactions are nil.

RECENT ADVANCES AND ITS IMPLICATIONS

The blunt tip needle recently introduced by Baheti DK[11] for these blocks (Celiac plexus block and lumbar sympathectomy) may further reduce the rate of iatrogenic complications such as injury to vessels, peritoneum and can be reduced.

The blunt tip needle used by author is a 20-gauge needle (locally made) is of stainless steel and can be repeated autoclaved.

REFERENCES

1. Kappis M. Erfahrungen mit lokalanaesthesia bei Bauch operationen. Verh Dtsch Ges Circ 1914;43:87.
2. Jones RR. A technique of injection of the splanchnic nerves with alcohol: Anesth. Analg 1957; 36:75.
3. Bride Baugh LD, Moore DC, Campbell DD. Management of upper abdominal cancer pain: Treatment with celiac plexus block with alcohol. JAMA 1964;190:877.
4. Jain S. The role of celiac plexus block in intractable upper abdominal pain. In Racz GB (Ed): Technique of neurolysis. Boston, Kluwer Academic, 1989, 161.
5. Brown DL, Bully CK, Quiel EC- Neurolytic celiac plexus block for pancreatic cancer pain. Anaesth. Analg 1987:66:869-73.
6. Thompson GE, Moore DC, Braidenbaugh LD. Abdominal pain and alcohol celiac plexus block Anesth. Analg 1977:56:1-5.
7. Baheti DK. Neurolytic coeliac plexus block (NCPB): A ten year review of 212 cases. Bombay Hospital Journal 2001;43:1.

8. Boas RA. Sympathetic blocks in clinical practice. In Stanton-Hicks M (Ed). International Anesthesia Clinics. Regional anesthesia: Advances in selected topics. Boston. Little Brown 1978;16:4.

9. Cousins MJ, Reeve TS, Glynn CJ, et al. Neurolytic sympathetic blockade: Duration of denervation and relief of rest pain. Anesth. Intensive care 1979;121-35,

10. P Prithviraj, et al. Celiac plexus block and neurolysis. Radiographic imaging for regional anesthesia and pain management. Churchill Livingston 2003; 164-74.

11. Baheti DK. Use of new modified needle with blunt tip for neurolytic sympathetic block in abdominal malignancies. Abstracts, 11th World Congress on Pain: I.A.S.P.Press 2005;489-90.

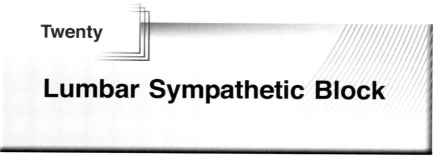

Twenty

Lumbar Sympathetic Block

DK Baheti

INTRODUCTION

Brunn and Mandl in 1924[1] first described the Sellheim's technique of Lumbar Sympathetic Plexus block.

INDICATIONS

Diagnosis and Treatment

- Vascular insufficiency due to
  - Peripheral vascular disease
  - Diabetes
  - Burger's disease
  - Raynaud's disease
  - Post vascular surgery
- Miscellaneous
  - Complex regional pain syndromes I and II
  - Herpes zoster
  - Stump pain
  - Phantom limb
  - Frost bite
  - Trench foot
  - Renal colic
  - Urogenital pain
  - Hyperhidrosis.

Contraindications

- Patient unable or unwilling to consent
- Known allergy to contrast
- Local infection
- Coagulopathy
- Uncooperative patient
- Pregnancy

- Concurrent use of anticoagulants
- Known systemic infection
- Coexisting disease producing significant CVS or respiratory compromise
- Immunosuppression.

Equipment/Types and Sizes of Needle

- Procedure room with C-Arm fluoroscopy or CT scan along with monitoring and resuscitation facility
- 26-gauge for skin infiltration and deep infiltration of local anesthetic
- 18-guage or 11 no. surgical blade for skin puncture to facilitate the insertion of blunt tip needle
- 20-guage 6" long blunt tip needle or 22-gauge 6" long needle
- Skin temperature monitor
- Emergency medications
- Needles: 3½ inch 25 G or 23 G needles
- Radiofrequency lesion generator.

Drugs and Concentration

- Inj. lignocaine- 2% (xylocard- preservative free)
- Inj. iohexol (omnipaque), a water soluble contrast
- Inj. bupivacaine 0.25%
- Inj. phenol in glycerine- 6 to10%.

Procedure

- Informed consent
- Patient preparation –I.V. and monitoring
- Antibiotics
- Prone position
- Square the endplates ipsilaterally under AP fluoroscopy.
- Identify the levels L2, L3 and L4.

POSITION AND LANDMARKS

Step 1 The patient is in prone position with a pillow under the pelvis to reverse to lumbar lordosis. The L2 to L4 spinous processes are felt and marking done. The point of needle entry is either four finger breadth or 6 to 8 cm from midline. Inj. 2% lidocaine about 10 cc intradermally and deep into the various layers in the direction of the needle. Then in case of blunt needle make a skin niche with 18-gauge hypodermic needle or with 11 no. surgical blade to facilitate the entry of blunt needle.

Step 2 The blunt tip needle is then directed to pass below and slightly medial to the inferior border of the transverse process at an angle of about 10° to the sagittal plane. It is advanced about 2 cm deep to the transverse process, where it should contact the side of the vertebral body. A slight decrease in the angle is made so as to allow the needle to slip past at a tangent to the lateral aspect of the vertebral body.

The position of the needle should be confirmed under fluoroscopy in lateral view and the tip of needle distance to the anterolateral surface of the vertebral body (Figs 20.1A and B).

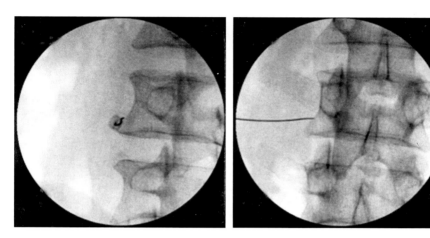

Figs 20.1A and B: Ideal needle positions for lumbar sympathetic blocks (A) Position of needle in lateral view; (B) Position of needle in AP view

Now confirm the loss of resistance. There should be no resistance to injection.

If there is resistance the tip is in the psoas fascia. Inject 1ml of contrast. In case the tip of needle is in psoas fascia then there will be a vacuolated retroperitoneal pattern (Fig. 20.2).

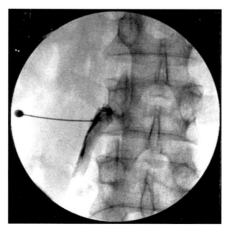

Fig. 20.2: Psoas injection vacuolated retroperitoneal pattern

Step 3   After confirmation of repeated negative aspiration, inject 4 to 5 cc of Inj. omnipaque 4 to 5 cc to confirm the spread of dye. Confirm the spread of dye in posterioanterior view the dye will hug vertically the spine. In lateral view the dye will spread along the anterior border of spine, save the images. The same procedure is repeated on opposite side (Figs 20.3A and B).

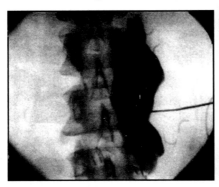 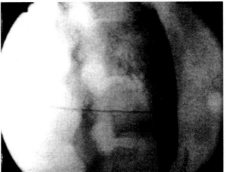

Fig. 20.3A: Spread of dye in AP view   **Fig. 20.3B:** Spread of dye lateral view

Step 4   For diagnostic block Inj. bupivacaine 0.25% 6 to 8 ml injected on each side. In case of neurolysis, Inj. phenol in oil 5 to 7cc on each side is injected. Warming up of phenol and flushing the needle with 1 to 2cc of normal saline will ease the injection of neurolytic agent (phenol).

Step 5   Before with drawing the needle put the stylet into it, to allow neurolytic agent to spill the desired area. Inject Inj. xylocaine 2% into the needle track while with drawing the needle. This will help to reduce the needle pain following the procedure.

Step 6   **Evidence of Sympatholysis**
- Vasodilatation in lower limbs
- Raised temperature in lower limbs
- Decreased edema.

Records

Permanent AP and lateral images should be obtained to document the final position of the needle and the extent of spread of the contrast.

Post-procedural Care

Step 7   The vital signs of the patient should be observed in the recovery for about 1 to 2 hours.

Problems

- Genitofemoral neuralgia up to 15%
- Intravascular injection
- Bleeding
- Hypotension.

Discharge Instructions

No Driving for that Day

- Patient should monitor and record the extent and duration of any relief that ensues
- Contact Doctor if headache, fever, chills, increased pain, paralysis or any other unusual symptoms
- Resume previous activities over a period of several days.

REFERENCE

1. Brunn F, Mandl F. Die paravertebrale injection Zur Bekaempfung visceraler Schmerzen. Wien Klin Aschsch 1924;37:511.

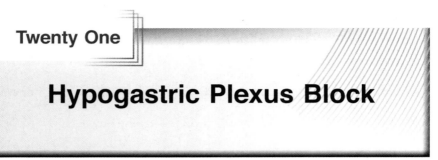

Twenty One

Hypogastric Plexus Block

DK Baheti, RP Gehdoo

INTRODUCTION

The superior hypogastric plexus lies in the retroperitoneal space anterior to the fifth lumbar vertebra left of the midline, just inferior to the aortic bifurcation. Its branches right and left and descends into the pelvis as the inferior hypogastric plexus which gives rise to the pelvic, middle rectal, vesicle, prostates, and uterovaginal plexus. Hypogastric plexus contains postganglionic sympathetic fibers and afferent visceral pain fibers. Many preganglionic parasympathetic fibers run independently and to the left of the superior hypogastric plexus. The inferior hypogastric plexus receives more parasympathetic fibers from the 2nd, 3rd, and 4th sacral levels.

Pelvic Innervations

The adnexal disorders pain is transmitted through the hypogastric plexus and celiac plexus along the sympathetic afferent fibers and enters the CNS at T10. Testicular pain transmitted through presacral ganglia along sympathetic afferents with the spermatic plexus and blood vessels to the CNS at the level of T10. Pain transmitted through presacral ganglion along sympathetic afferents through the spermatic plexus and blood vessels to the CNS at T10-11

Causes of Pelvic Pain

Endometriosis, carcinoma, of prostrate, uterus, cervix, rectum, sacrum, trauma, post inguinal herniorrhaphy (ilioinguinal, genitofemoral nerve trauma); chronic infection.

Indications

1. Chronic pain originating form pelvic viscera such as descending colon, rectum.
2. Tumors from uterus, ovary; endometriosis.
3. Excruating pain due to irritable bladder syndrome, interstitial cystitis, neurogenic bladder and bladder tumors.

4. Carcinoma of prostrate, testis, epididymisi
5. Bone tumors of sacrum.

Contraindications

- Patient unable or unwilling to consent
- Known allergy to contrast
- local infection
- Coagulopathy
- Uncooperative patient
- Pregnancy
- Concurrent use of anticoagulants
- Known systemic infection
- Coexisting disease producing significant CVS or respiratory compromise
- Immunosuppression.

Equipment/Types and Sizes of Needle

- Procedure room with C-arm fluoroscopy or CT scan along with monitoring and resuscitation facility.
- 26-gauge for skin infiltration and deep infiltration of local anesthetic.
- 18-guage needle or 11 no. surgical blade for skin puncture to facilitate the insertion of blunt tip needle.
- 20-guage 6″ long blunt tip needle or 22-gauge 6″ long needle.

Drugs and Concentration

- Inj. lignocaine- 2% (xylocard- preservative free)
- Inj. iohexol (omnipaque), a water soluble contrast
- Inj. bupivacaine 0.25%
- Inj. phenol in glycerine 6 to 10%.

PRE-OPERATIVE PREPARATION

Informed consent
Investigations such as complete blood count, bleeding time and clotting
An intravenous line
Monitoring of BP, SaO_2, and ECG
Antibiotic cover is necessary
Imaging facilities- fluoroscopy, ultrasound, or CT scan.

PROCEDURE

Lateral approach.[1]

Position and Landmarks

Step 1   The patient is in prone position with a pillow under the pelvis to reverse to lumbar lordosis (Fig. 21.1).

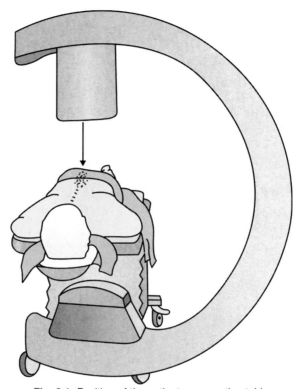

Fig. 2.1: Position of the patient on operation table

Step 2   The L4-L5 spinous processes are felt and marking done. Draw a line lateral to L4-L5 intervertebral space. The point of needle entry is either four finger breadth or 6 to 8 cm from midline. Inj. 2% lidocaine about 10 cc intradermally and deep into the various layers in the direction of the needle. If blunt needle is used then make a skin niche with 18-gauge hypodermic needle or with 11 no. surgical blade to facilitate the entry of blunt needle.

Step 3   The direction of needle should be approximately 45 degree medial and caudad to avoid the transverse process of L5 and ala of sacrum. In fluoroscopic lateral view confirm the tip of needle should be at anterior junction of L5-S1 vertabrae. Confirm position posterio-anterior view, the tip of needle must be no more than l cm from bony outline of L5-S1.

Step 4   After confirmation of repeated negative aspiration, Inject 4 to 5 cc of Inj. omnipaque 4 to 5 cc to confirm the spread of dye. Confirm the spread of dye in posterioanterior view the dye will hug vertically the spine. In lateral view the dye will spread along the anterior border of spine, save the images. The same procedure is repeated on opposite side (Figs 21.2 and 21.3).

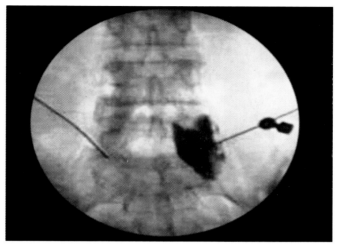

Fig. 21.2: Position of needle with spread of dye in AP view

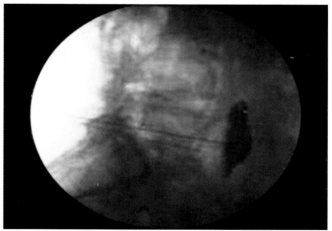

Fig. 21.3: Spread of dye in lateral view
Pictures courtesy: Dr Kailash Kothari and Dr C Das with permission

Step 5   For diagnostic block Inj. bupivacaine 0.25% 6 to 8 ml injected on each side. In case of neurolysis, Inj. phenol in oil 5 to 7 cc on each side is injected. Warming up of phenol and flushing the needle with 1 to 2 cc of normal saline will ease the injection of neurolytic agent (phenol).

Step 6   Before with drawing the needle put the stylet into it, to allow neurolytic agent to spill the desired area. Inject Inj. xylocaine 2%

into the needle track while with drawing the needle. This will help to reduce the needle pain following the procedure.

Step 7   The vital signs of the patient should be observed in the recovery for about 1-2 hours.

Other Approaches

Medial Approach

In this rotate the C-arm fluoroscope 15 degrees caudad so that x-ray beam will look into pelvis. As this view enlarges the space between L-5 transverse process, ala of sacrum and posterior anterior iliac spine.

Under local anesthesia under fluoroscopy mark the most inferior and lateral part of this bone free space. The direction of needle should be medial and slight caudad superior to the neural foramen. The tip of needle should be at the anterior edge of body of L5 vertebra. Repeat the same steps on opposite side.

After confirmation of negative aspiration inject 4 to 5 ml Inj. omnipaque on each side.

Evidence of Sympatholysis

* Vasodilatation in lower limbs
* Raised temperature in lower limbs
* Decreased edema
* Decreased pain with sympathetic mediated pain.

Records

Permanent AP and lateral images should be obtained to document the final position of the needle and the extent of spread of the contrast.

POST-PROCEDURAL CARE

The vital signs of the patient should be observed in the recovery for about 1 to 2 hours.

Problems

* Intravascular injection
* Bleeding
* Hypotension.

Discharge Instructions

No Driving for that Day

* Patient should monitor and record the extent and duration of any relief that ensues

- Contact Doctor if headache, fever, chills, increased pain, paralysis or any other unusual symptoms
- Resume previous activities over a period of several days.

REFERENCE

1. Plancarte R, Amescua C, Patt RB, Aldrete JA. Superior hypogastric plexus block for pelvic cancer pain. Anesthesiology 1990;73:23.

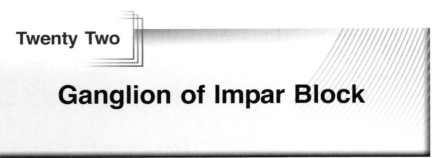

Twenty Two

Ganglion of Impar Block

DK Baheti

INTRODUCTION

The ganglion of Impar is also known as Ganglion of Walther[1] and is the last ganglion of the sympathetic trunk. It is single ganglion formed with fusion of two ganglions of both sides and located retroperitoneally at level of sacrococcygeal junction that marks termination of the paired paravertebral chains. This receives fibers from the lumbar and sacral portions of sympathetic and parasympathetic nervous system.

Indications

Pain originating either from pelvic viscera or sympathetically maintained pain in the perineum is effective managed by ganglion of impar block. The pain may be vague, burning or localized in perineum.

Equipment/Types and Sizes of Needle (Fig. 22.1)

- Procedure room with C-arm fluoroscopy or CT scan along with monitoring and resuscitation facility.
- 26-gauge for skin infiltration and deep infiltration of local anesthetic.
- 18-gauge needle or 11 no. surgical blade for skin puncture to facilitate the insertion of blunt tip needle.
- 22-gauge 3½" long spinal needle.

Drugs and Concentration

- Inj. lignocaine 2% (xylocard- preservative free).
- Iohexol (omnipaque) water soluble dye.
- Inj. bupivacaine 0.25%.
- Inj. phenol in glycerine 6 to 10%.

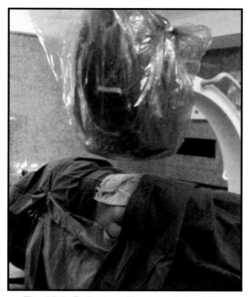

Fig. 22.1: Patient position lateral decubitus

Procedure

Pre-operative Preparation

1. Informed consent.
2. Investigations such as complete blood count, bleeding time and clotting time.
3. Procedure to be done in procedure room or in operation theater.
4. Monitoring of BP, SaO_2, and ECG is mandatory.
5. I.V. access.
6. Antibiotic cover.
7. Imaging facility- C-arm fluoroscopy.

LATERAL POSITION APPROACH – ANOCOCCYGEAL OR TRANS-SACROCOCCYGEAL APPROACH

Position and Landmarks

Step 1   Patient in lateral decubitus position with hip flexed. C-arm placed at gluteal region focusing on sacrococcygeal bone.
Inj. xylocaine 1% 3 to 5 cc at the level of anococcygeal ligament, i.e. midway between tip of coccyx and anus.

Step 2   Under fluoroscopy put an artery forceps just below sacrococcygeal ligament.

Step 3 Infiltrate Inj. 2% lignocaine 4 to 5 cc deep upto sacrococcygeal ligament (Fig. 22.2).

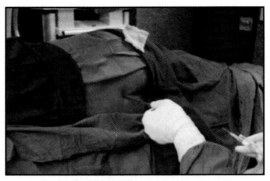

Fig. 22.2: Entry point for needle

Step 4 Push 22-gauge 3.5 inch needle directly into the retroperitoneal space. Confirm the position of needle under fluoroscopy (Fig. 22.3).

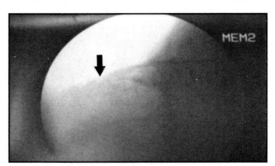

Fig. 22.3: Needle in AP view

Step 5 After repeated negative aspiration inject 3 to 4 cc Inj. omnipaque to confirm the spread of dye (Fig. 22.4).

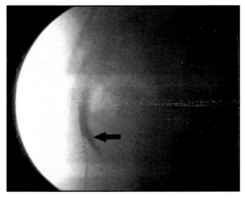

Fig. 22.4: Spread of dye lateral view

Step 6 For diagnostic block Inj. bupivacaine 0.25% 6 to 8 ml injected on each side.

In case of neurolysis, Inj. phenol in oil 5 to 7 cc on each side is injected. Warming up of phenol and flushing the needle with 1 to 2 cc of normal saline will ease the injection of neurolytic agent (phenol).

Step 7 Before with drawing of needle insert the stylet into it, to allow neurolytic agent to spill the desired area. Inject Inj. xylocaine 2% into the needle track while with drawing the needle. This will help to reduce the needle pain following the procedure.

Step 8 The vital signs of the patient should be observed in the recovery for about 1 to 2 hours.

Another Technique

Another technique is as follows:

Bent the spinal needle[2] according to the curvature of coccyx, and introduce the needle in midline and care to be taken not to puncture rectal wall. It is advisable to introduce one finger into the rectum and guide the needle slowly.

Confirm the tip of the needle under fluoroscopy. After repeated negative aspiration inject Inj. omnipaque 1 to 2 cc. Confirm the spread of the dye in lateral and anterioposterior view. Save these pictures for documentation.

Contraindications

1. Anticoagulation therapy or suffer from congenital abnormalities of coagulation.
2. Antiblastic cancer therapy.
3. The local skin infection at needle entry point or intra abdominal infection and sepsis, intestinal obstruction.

REFERENCES

1. Warfield CA, Bajwa ZH. Principles and practice of pain medicine, New Delhi Tata McGraw Publishing Company limited 2004;1:366.
2. Plancarte R, Amescua C, Patt R, Allende S. Pre sacral blockade of ganglion of Walther (ganglion impar) [Abstract] Anesthesiology 1990;73;A 751.

Section F

Spine and Back

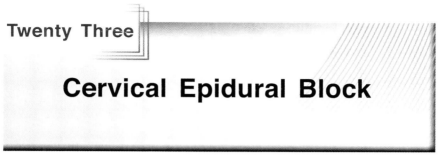

Twenty Three

Cervical Epidural Block

H Bram

OVERVIEW

Cervical epidural injections, whether by translaminar or transforaminal approach, are common techniques employed by interventional pain specialists. These injections can be used for therapeutic or diagnostic purposes. A physician who performs these injections should be well versed and trained in lumbar epidural injections prior to attempting injections into the cervical epidural space.

ANATOMY

The epidural space extends from the foramen magnum down to the sacrococcygeal junction. The epidural space is bounded posteriorly by the ligamentum flavum, laterally by the pedicles and intervertebral foramen, and anteriorly by the posterior longitudinal ligament. The epidural space contains fat, veins, arteries, connective and lymphatic tissue.[1] Nerve roots traverse the epidural space as they exit through their respective neural foramina.

Flexion of the head increases the epidural space at the C7-T1. It is important to note, for translaminar injections, that the epidural space narrows above the C7-T1 segment increasing the potential for dural puncture or spinal cord injury.

Indications

Cervical epidural injections are commonly employed to treat cervical radiculopathy, cervical spondylosis, and neck pain. They can also be used to treat pain emanating from cancer, such as a compressive lesion on a nerve root. Less commonly they can be employed to treat symptoms related to acute herpes zoster or a vaso-occlusive disorder such as Raynaud's disease or frostbite.[2]

Diagnostic transforaminal / selective root injections may be requested by a surgeon, prior to surgery, in an attempt to isolate a potential pain-generating segment.

Contraindications

The absolute contraindications for performing epidural injections are coagulopathy, bleeding disorders, patient refusal, and an infection at the intended needle insertion site.[3] For transforaminal injections inability to inject contrast, secondary to dye allergy, would also be an absolute contraindication.

There are several relative contraindications: systemic infection, allergy to injectate (if there is not a substitute for the intended injectate, i.e. local anesthetic) and anatomic variations or postsurgical changes that alter the anatomy in which the injection could result in an adverse outcome. A patient with a physiologic disorder, such as a very brittle diabetic for epidural steroid injection or cardiopulmonary compromise, e.g. patient with phrenic nerve paralysis who is unable to lie supine or in a lateral decubitus position.

Equipment

Transforaminal epidural steroid injections can result in potential life-threatening situations. Thus, certain equipment needs to be available for this procedure, whether it is performed in a hospital setting, free-standing, ambulatory suite, or in the office. The procedure room needs to have suction, oxygen source, airway equipment, emergency drugs, and monitoring equipment (Fig. 23.1). The Author always has intravenous access prior to starting the procedure.

If one is performing a cervical epidural steroid injection, using the translaminar approach and is planning on injecting local anesthetic into the epidural space, the same equipment, including intravenous access, needs to be available, as for a transforaminal injection, in case inadvertent subarachnoid or subdural injection should occur.

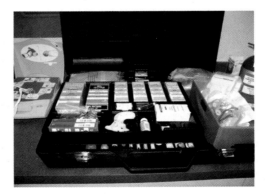

Fig. 23.1: Emergency drugs, oxygen, AED

Equipment for Translaminar Epidural Steroids

For proper visualization, fluoroscopy is required. A C-arm, which has the ability to provide a clear image and can be positioned into multiple angles.

- Antiseptic solution such as betadine with applicator sticks or Dura Prep® and sterile drape
- 5 cc syringe – for the steroid/preservative free saline or local anesthetic
- 3 cc syringe - for contrast
- 5 cc syringe – for local anesthetic for skin anesthesia
- 5 cc loss of resistance syringe either glass or plastic
- 20 Gz Tuohy or Huber needle 10 cm in length
- 25 Gz or 27 Gz 5/8 inch to 1 inch spinal needle for skin anesthesia
- 5 cc to 10 cc of 1% lidocaine for skin anesthesia
- Nonionic contrast, such as omnipaque 240® or Isovue M200®
- Triamcinolone 40 mg/cc or betamethasone 6 mg/cc.
- Preservative free saline
- 1% preservative free lidocaine or 0.25% bupivacaine.

If the patient is allergic to the nonionic dye, for translaminar epidural steroid injections, the Author has substituted 1 to 2 cc of gadolinium (Magnevist®). Although acceptable for translaminar epidural steroid injections, this dye is very faint and is not appropriate as a substitute for transforaminal epidural injections.

Equipment for Transforaminal Injections

For proper visualization, fluoroscopy is required. A C-arm, which has the ability to provide a clear image and can be positioned into multiple angles.
- Sterile prep solution either betadine or DuraPrep®
- Sterile drape (the Author prefers a clear fenestrated drape so that he is able to visualize the patient's face)
- 25 Gz or 27 Gz needle, 5/8 to 1 inch for skin anesthesia
- 1% lidocaine for skin anesthesia
- Three 3 cc syringes
- Three extension tubings
- 25-Gauge 2.5 inch short bevel needle
- Preservative free 1% or 2% preservative free lidocaine
- Nonionic contrast – Omnipaque 240® or Isovue-M 200®
- Triamcinolone 40 mg/cc, betamethasone 6 mg/cc or dexamethasone 10 mg/cc.

TECHNIQUE FOR TRANSLAMINAR EPIDURAL INJECTIONS

As with any interventional technique, the patient should be examined and an appropriate history obtained prior to the procedure. The risk should be discussed, which include, but are not limited to; allergic reaction, bleeding, infection, nerve injury or damage, and postdural puncture headache. In experienced hands, the highest risk is postdural puncture headache, which is less than 1%. After the risks and benefits are discussed, consents should be signed.

If the patient is having the translaminar epidural injection under strict local anesthetic with no local anesthesic being injected into the epidural space, intravenous access is not mandatory. If the patient is receiving local anesthetic into the epidural space, then intravenous access needs to be obtained.

The patient is brought into the procedure room and placed in a prone position with a pillow under the chest with the neck flexed. The arms can be placed at the patient's sides or placed above the head (Fig. 23.2). If lateral X-ray is being considered, during the procedure, the arms will need to be at the sides. An antiseptic solution, such as betadine or DuraPrep® is applied and strict aseptic technique should be employed. If sedation is being administered, the patient should only receive light sedation and the physician should be able to maintain verbal contact with the patient throughout the procedure. If the patient, while receiving light sedation, becomes verbally unresponsive, then the procedure should be stopped and the physician should wait until the sedation dissipates to the point where he can resume verbal communication. Failure to be able to speak with the patient during the procedure increases the patient's risk.

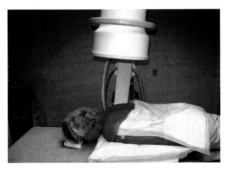

Fig. 23.2: Patient position for cervical epidural injection

The C7-T1 interspace is identified under radiological guidance (Fig. 23.3). The C-arm is placed in AP plane with a slight craniad or caudad tilt. The skin is anesthetized with 1% or 2% lidocaine. A 5/8 to 1 inch needle can be used for skin anesthesia.

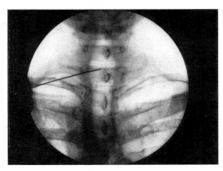

Fig. 23.3: Pointer at C7-T1 interspace

After the skin is anesthetized with local, a 20-gauge Tuohy needle is inserted until contact with the lamina of T1 with the needle in the midline or just lateral the midline. This provides the physician with an idea of the depth to the epidural space. The needle is then withdrawn slightly and the loss-of-resistance syringe is attached. The needle is then advanced craniad off the lamina and using loss-of-resistance technique, the epidural space is located. After gentle aspiration for cerebrospinal fluid and blood, 1 to 2 cc of nonionic contrast is injected, which should show epidural spread (Fig. 23.4). Lateral X-rays can be used to confirm needle position, however, with the patient in the prone position lateral radiographs are sometimes difficult to obtain secondary to obstruction from the patient's shoulders. The operator should evaluate for rapid run off of dye, which would be indicative of vascular uptake and if this occurs, the needle should be withdrawn and re-inserted

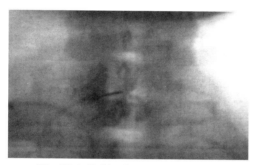

Fig. 23.4: Epidural spread of contrast

into the epidural space again using loss-of-resistance technique. The practitioner may also notice contrast that appears as a band or streak and does not diffuse across the midline like typical epidural spread (Fig. 23.5). This signifies that the needle is superficial to the epidural space. Epidural spread is normal or it can be extended several segments above the insertion site at C7-T1. It is not recommended to go above the C7-T1 using intralaminar approach because the risk of spinal cord trauma is higher above this segment since the epidural space narrows above C7-T1.

After confirming needle position, steroid solution, i.e. 80 mg of triamcinolone mixed with 3 cc of preservative-free normal saline can be injected for treatment of cervical radiculopathy. If local anesthetic is desired, 0.5 to 1% lidocaine 3 cc can be injected or other low concentration local anesthetic. If local anesthetic is used, this should be always with extreme caution. If inadvertent spinal or subdural injection can occur, then the patient can have profound hemodynamic shifts with marked hypotension. Any physician administering local anesthetic into the epidural space needs to be aware of the potential complications and be able to provide airway and hemodynamic support.

The epidural needle should be cleared, if steroid is injected, by reinserting the stylet, after the needle is withdrawn from the epidural space or by putting

1 mL to 2 cc of air through the needle so that you do not leave a potential steroid tract. The patient is then observed as per office or surgical center protocol and discharged to home if in stable condition.

Complications – Translaminar Epidural Injections

The potential complications from translaminar epidural steroid injections are not very common. The most common side effect from epidural injections is postdural puncture headache, which can be managed by conservative means. Other potential complications include nerve injury and spinal cord trauma. It cannot be over emphasized that these injections should never be performed with heavy sedation in which the patient cannot respond verbally to the pain interventionalist. The patient should be able to react to painful stimuli and if intravenous analgesics are employed they should be used very judiciously. If local anesthetic is employed, the physician needs to be able to deal with the possibility of subarachnoid or subdural injection, which again could result in marked hypotension. Vascular absorption of medication, infection and allergic reaction to medication can also occur.

Transforaminal Injections Technique

The patient, like translaminar epidurals, is evaluated prior to the procedure. Risks are again discussed with the patient, which include, but are not limited to; bleeding, infection, nerve injury, postdural puncture headache, potential for spinal anesthetic, and paralysis. This procedure can result in permanent neurological damage and even death, and only physicians who are experienced in interventional techniques should perform this procedure.

The patient is brought into the procedure room and placed in a supine position (Fig. 23.5). (This procedure can also be performed in the oblique or lateral decubitus position, however the following description will focus with the patient in the supine position). The patient's neck is prepped using strict aseptic technique. If sedation is given, only light sedation should be used and the physician should always be able to maintain verbal contact with the patient.

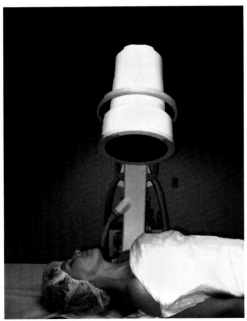

Fig. 23.5: Patient position for transforaminal epidural steroid injection on the left side

The fluoroscopy unit is placed into an oblique plane and a caudad tilt may be applied in order to best visualize the desired foramen. The first foramen visualized is C2-C3 with the C3 nerve exist this foramen (Fig. 23.6). The lower half of the posterior wall of the foramen is formed by the superior articular process. The desired target is the mid portion of the posterior wall, which corresponds to the upper portion of the superior articular process (Fig. 23.7). The needle will need to contact the anterior half of the superior articular process. After skin anesthesia with 1 to 2% local anesthetic, a 25 Gz 2.5 inch short bevel spinal needle is directed under fluoroscopic guidance down to the bony contact of the upper portion of the superior articular process. This should be done either under continuous fluoroscopic guidance or with small movements of the needle and then checking the needle position. The needle should not stray into the foramen. The patient at times will experience some pain into the neck and shoulder; however, if paresthesias occur in the arm, the needle needs to be redirected. Once the superior articular process is

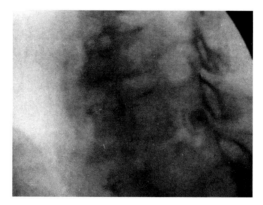

Fig. 23.6: Needle C3 foramen lat. view

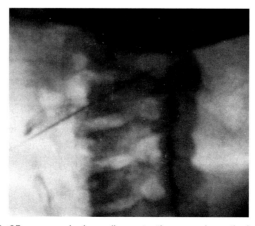

Fig. 23.7: 25-gauge spinal needle contacting superior articular process

contacted, the needle should be slightly withdrawn and re-directed anteriorly over the bone into the foramen (Fig. 23.8). The depth past the superior articular process into the foramen is only a few millimeters and position should be checked on AP fluoroscopy. The needle should not cross beyond the midline of the facet pillars (Fig. 23.9). Once the needle has been placed and after negative aspiration for cerebrospinal fluid and blood, 1 cc of nonionic

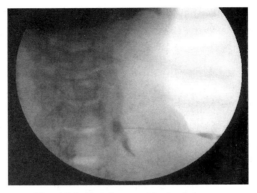

Fig. 23.8: Needle entering the foramen

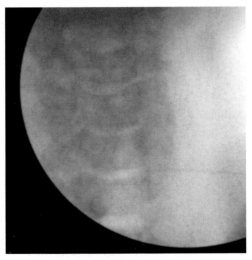

Fig. 23.9: AP view of needle placement

contrast, i.e. omnipaque 240® or isovue-M 200® is injected, under live fluoroscopy, and one should visualize spread down the nerve root and flow into the epidural space (Figs 23.10 and 23.11). If there is quick absorption of the contrast on live fluoroscopy with superior spread, the needle may be in the vertebral artery. Rapid absorption with spread over the anterior surface

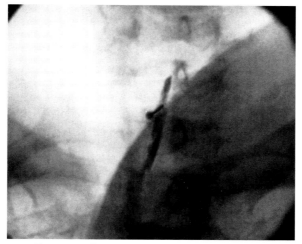

Fig. 23.10: Contrast in epidural space in AP view

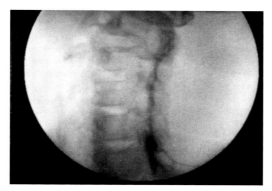

Fig. 23.11: Oblique view of contrast in the epidual space

of vertebral body could signify flow into the anterior spinal artery (The Author aborts the procedure if arterial flow is observed). Subarchnoid flow of contrast may also be observed in which case the needle will need to be repositioned. If adequate dye spread is noted, then 1% or 2% lidocaine can be injected into the epidural space and 1 cc should suffice.

If steroids are used, the physician should wait to make sure that intravascular or subarachnoid absorption of the local anesthetic does not occur. If there are no adverse side effects from the local anesthetic injection, epidural steroids can be injected, which can be 20 to 40 mg of triamcinolone, 6 to 12 mg of betamethasone, or 10 to 12 mg of dexamethasone.

The needle is withdrawn from the epidural space and cleared by inserting the stylet back into the needle so as not to leave a steroid tract. The patient is observed for an appropriate period of time and then discharged to home.

Complications – Transforaminal Epidural Injections

The potential complications from transforaminal cervical epidural steroid injections include: postdural puncture headache, allergic reaction, infection, injury to a nerve root or potential insertion of the needle into the spinal cord and intravascular injection of medication. The most serious potential complications are spinal cord injury and arterial injection of particulate steroid resulting in neurological damage or even death.

The physician also has to be aware that local anesthetics injected, even in small amounts, if inadvertently placed into the cerebral spinal fluid can result in total spinal anesthesia.

REFERENCES

1. Bogduk, Nikolai. Practice guidelines for spinal diagnostic and treatment procedures. San Francisco, CA: International Spine Intervention Society 2004;244.
2. McGraw, Kevin J. Interventional radiology of the spine. Totowa, New Jersey: Humana Press, 2004;127-8.
3. Raj P Prithvi. Radiographic imaging for regional anesthesia and pain management. Philadelphia, PA: Churchill Livingstone, 2003;101, table 16-1.

Twenty Four

Cervical Facet, Median Branch Blocks

H Bram

Cervical facet injections and cervical medial branch blocks are primarily diagnostic injections. Cervical facet injections can be used for therapeutic purposes, but in general are for diagnostic purposes. These injections are used primarily to isolate the pain-causing generators. The physician, if he is able to locate the painful segment can potentially offer the patient an ablative procedure, such as radiofrequency rhizotomy, to provide more profound and longer-lasting technique. There is not an advantage in performing a cervical facet intra-articular injection over a cervical medial branch block. Furthermore, there is a higher risk of potential complications from an intra-articular injection.

ANATOMY

The cervical facet joints are composed of a superior facet articulating with an inferior facet process. The cervical facet joint is innervated by the medial branch of the dorsal ramus. Each facet joint has dual innervation: the medial branch at the level of the joint and is also supplied by the medial branch from the level above. Thus, at C4-5 this facet joint is innervated by the medial branch from C4-5 and also from the medial branch at C3-4. This has important clinical applications in that when performing a medial branch block, for diagnostic information, 2 levels need to be anesthetized to evaluate a specific facet joint as a potential pain generator.

The medial branches course along the posteriolateral and anteriolateral articular pillars. The C4, C5 and C6 traverse the midportion of the articular pillars. The C7 medial branch courses along the superior portion of the articular pillar.[1]

At C3, there are again 2 medial branches: the larger, superior medial branch, also known as the Third Occipital Nerve and the deep medial branch. The Third Occipital Nerve runs, with some variation, across the C2-3 facet line or just inferior to the facet joint line margin.

The deep medial branch runs inferior and parallel to the third occipital nerve at the C3 articular pillar.[2]

INDICATIONS

Cervical facet and cervical medial branch blocks are predominately for diagnostic evaluation of cervicogenic headaches, neck and shoulder pain.

CONTRAINDICATIONS

The absolute contraindication for this procedure is patient's refusal, patient with coagulation or bleeding abnormalities, and infection at the injection site. The relative contraindications would be distorted anatomy, in which the operator will not be able to deposit the medication into the target region and systemic infection.

EQUIPMENT-CERVICAL FACET AND CERVICAL MEDIAL BRANCH BLOCK

The equipment required is the same for both facet and medial branch blocks.
*   An antiseptic solution such as betadine or DuraPrep
*   Sterile drape
*   22 Gz or 25 Gz needles 3.5 inch for regular sized adults and 5 inch needles for larger patients
*   1% or 2% lidocaine for skin anesthesia
*   5 mL or 10 cc syringes
*   Sterile tubing
*   0.5 % bupivacaine, 0.75% ropivacaine or 0.5% ropivacaine
*   Triamcinolone 40 mg/cc or celestone 6 mg/cc
*   Nonionic contrast- Omnipaque 240® or Isovue M-200®
*   C-arm for fluoroscopic guidance.

TECHNIQUE- CERVICAL MEDIAL BRANCH BLOCK

Consent is obtained from the patient after appropriate history and physical examination is performed. The patient is brought into the procedure room and placed prone on the table with arms at the side and pillow under the chest. The patient is prepped using antiseptic solution and strict aseptic technique. For the cervical medial branch blocks, the head is turned away from the target side (Fig. 24.1). Thus if one is working on the left

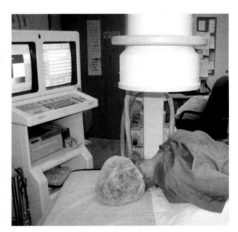

Fig. 24.1: Position of patient and C-arm

side, the head is turned to the right to give better visualization of the articular pillars as identified by the concavities (Fig. 24.2).

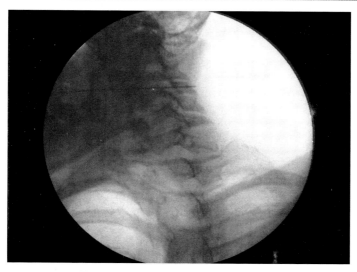

Fig. 24.2: Needles lateral to articular pillar

The C-arm is in AP plane and rotated slightly caudad to give sharp visualization of the concavities. Skin is anesthetized with local anesthetic immediately lateral to the articular pillars. The needles are inserted aiming at the lateral most aspect of the posterior surface of the bone.

After bony contact, the needle is withdrawn and moved slightly laterally immediately adjacent to concavity (Fig. 24.3).

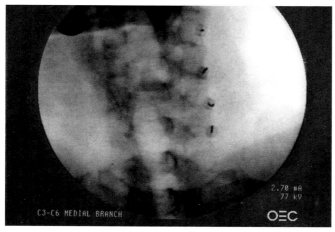

Fig. 24.3: Needles in AP view

Lateral X-rays are taken and the needles should be positioned within the midportion of the articular pillar (Fig. 24.4).

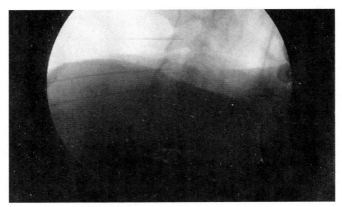

Fig. 24.4: Needles in align to articular pillars

The C-arm needs to be adjusted to align the articular pillars or trapezoid for a true lateral view (Fig. 24.5).

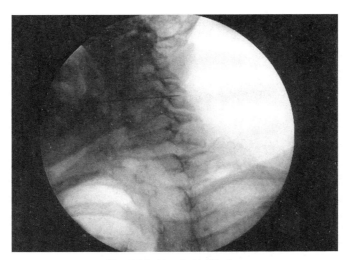

Fig. 24.5: Needle in AP view

Once the needles are in place, 0.3 mL to 1 cc of local anesthetic, i.e. 0.5% bupivacaine is injected. For strictly diagnostic purposes only local anesthetic should be injected and for diagnostic and therapeutic purposes, 1 mg / cc of celestone or 10 mg/cc of triamcinolone can be added into the solution. The needles are retracted and cleared by inserting the stylet back into the needle so as not to leave a steroid track. The patient is discharged to home after an appropriate period of time for postprocedural observation.

For C3 or Third Occipital Nerve block, because of variable location, one needle should be inserted to the midportion of the C2-3 facet line, with a second and third needle being placed immediately superior and inferior to the C2-3 facet line.[1] For C3-6 medial branches the needles need to be inserted in the midportion of the articular process. For C7 medial branch block, the needle should be inserted along the superior portion of the articular pillar.

COMPLICATIONS

The risk from cervical medial branch block injections is in general, quite low. The patient may experience temporary dizziness or ataxia from relaxation of the posterior cervical musculature in the cervical spine and this is a temporary affect, which resolves when the local anesthetic dissipates. The patient may also potentially experience paresthesias in the arms or weakness in the arms from anterior spread of the local anesthetic. Vascular absorbtion, allergic reaction and infection are also potential complications.

CERVICAL FACET - INTRAARTICULAR TECHNIQUE

The patient is brought into the procedure room and placed in prone position. A pillow is placed under the chest and the neck is flexed and turned away from the affected side.

The patient is prepped and draped using strict sterile technique.

The target facet joint is identified on fluoroscopic view with the C-arm. Caudad tilt is placed on the C-arm in the anterior-posterior plane for sharp visualization of the target joint.

The skin is anesthetized with local anesthetic, such as 1 % lidocaine. A 22 or 25-guage spinal needle is inserted towards the inferior aspect of the

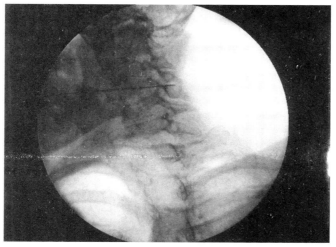

Fig. 24.6: Needle position in oblique view

facet joint towards the mid position of the joint (Fig. 24.6). The needle, after it strikes the bone is then withdrawn and re-directed superiorly to enter the joint. Lateral X-ray is used to confirm that the needle is within the substance of the joint. Care must be taken that the needle is within the substance of the joint and does not extend through the joint for spinal cord trauma could occur. After negative aspiration, the interventionist can inject a small amount of nonionic contrast, 0.3 cc of omnipaque 240 or isovue-M 200 into the joint to confirm that dye stays within the joint and does not spread into the epidural or intrathecal region. If dye flow is suitable, then 0.5 cc of local anesthetic can be injected, such as 0.5% ropivacaine or bupivicaine with 10 mg of triamcinolone. The needle is withdrawn from the space and stylette is re-inserted to clear the needle. The patient is observed for an appropriate amount of time and discharged to home.

COMPLICATION

Intraarticular cervical facet injections can result in spinal cord injury, nerve injury, vascular absorption, allergic reaction, infection and epidural or spinal anesthesia.

REFERENCES

1. Bogduk, Nikolai. Practice guidelines for spinal diagnostic and treatment procedures. San Francisco, CA: International Spine Intervention Society 2004;124-5.
2. Waldman, Steven D. Interventional pain management (2nd Edn). Philadelphia, PA: WB. Saunders Company 2001;458.

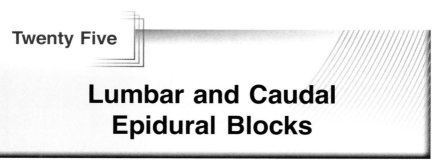

Twenty Five

Lumbar and Caudal Epidural Blocks

S Bakshi, GW Abrahamsen

INTRODUCTION

Epidural steroid injections are the placement of steroids into the epidural space. They were first described in 1953 and epidural steroids have been administered to millions of patients for the treatment of axial and radicular back pain. Traditionally, these injections were performed with a "blind approach" (without fluoroscopy) and lacked target specificity and contrast spread to confirm needle placement into the epidural space. With the advent and use of fluoroscopy the transforaminal approach became widespread, with the thought that epidural steroids would be more effective if they were delivered more accurately to the site of pathology.[1-4]

At the present time, the efficacy of epidural steroid injections remains controversial. Only six prospective, blinded, randomized, controlled trials reporting the efficacy of epidural steroids have been performed. Two reported significant improvement of symptoms[5,6] and four did not.[7-10] A meta-analysis of the epidural steroid injection literature from 1996 to 1993 revealed a 14% positive treatment effect over placebo.[11] However, the earlier studies were again performed with "blind" techniques.

The basis behind the use of epidural steroid injections is that chemical mediators are released from a disc after injury to that disc. This results in the release of phospholipase A2 (PLA2) from the nucleus pulposus into the epidural space.[12] PLA2 is an enzyme found in high concentrations in disc material. PLA2 is highly inflammatogenic and propagates an inflammatory cascade with the liberation of arachidonic acid with inflammatory responses via leukotrienes and prostaglandins.[13] Epidural steroids act by blocking PLA2 activity and can exert an anesthetic like activity by blocking nociceptive C-fiber conduction.[14] This effect is reversed when the corticosteroid is removed, suggesting a direct membrane effect. Glucocorticoid receptor sites have also been located on norepinephrine and 5-hydroxytryptamine neurons within the dorsal horn substantia gelatinosa.[15,16]

ANATOMY

The epidural space lies between the osseoligamentous structures lining the vertebral canal and the dural membrane surrounding the spinal cord and the nerve roots.[17]

The anterior epidural space is bordered anteriorly by the vertebral body, intervertebral disc, and posterior longitudinal ligament and posteriorly by the thecal sac. The posterior epidural space is bordered anteriorly by the thecal sac and posteriorly by the ligamentum flavum and the laminae. Each spinal nerve exists within an intervertebral foramen, bordered anteriorly by the vertebral body and the disc, posteriorly by the facet joint, and superiorly and inferiorly by the pedicles of the adjacent vertebrae.

Evaluation

Evaluation of a patient with back pain should begin with a detailed history and physical examination. Patients will often complain of lower back pain with radicular symptoms to the lower extremities, including pain, numbness, paresthesiae, or weakness. Patients will often also describe symptoms consistent with neurogenic claudication. Physical examination may reveal paresthesiae in a dermatomal distribution; weakness in a myotomal distribution; and a positive straight-leg raise.

Imaging studies should be performed including plain film radiographs and MRI or CT scan to confirm a diagnosis that will benefit from epidural steroid injections. Electrodiagnostic signs of radiculopathy may be helpful, but are not an absolute prerequisite to epidural injections.

Indications

The main clinical indications for epidural steroid injections include: Disc degeneration or herniation, spinal nerve root compression, spinal nerve root inflammation, and spinal stenosis. Correlating the distribution of the patients pain with the imaging study findings, the clinician can then decide which epidural technique, level, and side of spine at which the injection should be performed to achieve maximum benefit.

Epidural steroid injections should then be performed if the patient has a diagnosed cause of radiculopathy, has not responded to non-surgical conservative measures, and whose pain is likely to have an inflammatory basis.

Contraindications

Absolute contraindications to epidural steroid injections include patients who are unwilling to consent to the procedure, evidence of an untreated infection at the site of the injection, pregnancy, and bleeding diathesis. Relative contraindications are known allergy to the medications and dye administered, concurrent use of anticoagulant medication, known systemic infection, immunosuppression, severe respiratory or cardiovascular compromise, and anatomic, congenital or surgical changes preventing safe administration of medication into the epidural space. If the patient has a known allergy to the medications used for the procedure, pre-medication may then be required depending on the severity of the allergic reaction.

Equipment/Supplies

When performing epidural injections a C-arm fluoroscope is required for precise needle placement and visualization of flow of contrast. The equipment and supplies needed include: Tuohy epidural needles, 18 or 20-gauge 3.5 inch (interlaminar), spinal needle, 22 or 25-gauge 5 inch short bevel needle (transforaminal), 25-gauge 1.5 inch needle for administration of local anesthetic, syringe 5 mL. 10 mL glass or plastic syringe (for interlaminar approach using "loss of resistance technique"), 10 mL plastic syringe, 3 mL syringe for injection of contrast, connection tubing, sterile gloves, drapes, gowns, and povidone-iodine or chlorhexidine prep. Typically, the supplies can be packaged in a custom epidural tray. Most patients also require intravenous access. In some cases I.V. sedation is used. Physiological monitoring should also be used throughout the procedure.

Medications

Medications used for epidural steroid injections vary but include: preservative free sterile saline, water soluble, non-ionic radiographic contrast medium (isovue or omnipaque), local anesthetic (lidocaine 1-2% or bupivicaine (0.125 - 0.5%), and a corticosteroid preparation (triamcinolone 20-80 mg, betamethasone 6-18 mg, depomedrol 20-80 mg or dexamethasone).[18,19]

Common volumes used for the injectate include: Interlaminar approach: total volume 6 to 8 mL, Transforaminal approach: total volume 2 mL, and Caudal approach: total volume 10 to 15 mL. The clinician will then combine 1 to 2 mL of corticosteroid with local anesthetic or normal saline to achieve the desired volume.

Techniques

The interlaminar approach, both midline and paramedian, involves insertion of an epidural needle midway between the laminae of the adjacent vertebrae, whereas the transforaminal approach involves insertion of a spinal needle into the superior portion of an intervertebral foramen just inferior to the pedicle.

Procedure

Interlaminar Approach

After informed consent is obtained, patient is placed prone on the fluoroscopy table. It is advisable to place a small pillow under the lower abdomen to open up the interlaminar space. At this point the skin is prepped and draped in a sterile fashion.

After carefully identifying the appropriate interlaminar space that you want to enter using fluoroscopy, make a skin mark over the lamina below the target interspace. The skin and subcutaneous tissues are now anesthetized using 1% lidocaine.

A 20-gauge Tuohy needle is now advanced to the lamina. It is preferable to contact the superior border of the lower lamina so that you have perception of the appropriate depth. The needle can now be walked off the lamina till it is felt to enter the ligamentum flavum. At this point attach a "loss of resistance" syringe to the needle. Depending on operator preference you can either use saline or air for the loss of resistance technique. Carefully advance the needle in small increments till you feel the loss of resistance on entering the epidural space. Once the epidural space is entered 1 to 2 cc of radio contrast dye is injected and the dye spread is visualized under continuous fluoroscopy in the AP position. The C-arm is now rotated to the lateral position and appropriate dye spread is reconfirmed in the lateral position. The dye spread should be in the epidural space and there should be no intravascular or intrathecal flow patterns. It is advisable to save the hard copy of the dye spread patterns in both AP and lateral views (Figs 25.1A to F).

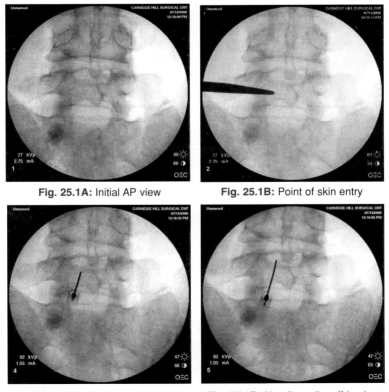

Fig. 25.1A: Initial AP view   **Fig. 25.1B:** Point of skin entry

Fig. 25.1C: Needle headed to lamina   **Fig. 25.1D:** Needle walks off lamina

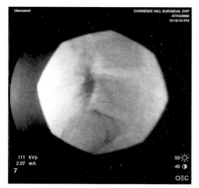 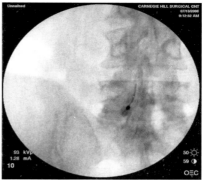

Fig. 25.1E: Reconfirm position on lat.   **Fig. 25.1F:** AP view of dye spread

Transforaminal Approach

After informed consent is obtained, patient is placed prone on the fluoroscopy table. Skin is prepped and draped in a sterile fashion.

After starting in the AP position, the C-arm is rotated slightly in an oblique fashion, so that the typical Scotty dog picture can be visualized. The initial target is the 6 o' clock position of the pedicle. A skin mark is placed directly over this point. Skin and subcutaneous tissues are then anesthetized using 1% lidocaine. A 22 or 25-gauge 5 inch short bevel needle is then advanced under fluoroscopic guidance towards the target point. The needle position is then checked initially in the AP position and subsequently in the lateral position to ensure that the tip of the needle is finally in optimum position. At this point in the AP view the tip of the needle should lie just below the mid-point of the pedicle and should not cross the facet joint line. In the lateral view the needle tip should lie in the posterior superior quadrant of the neural foramen. At this point once the needle is felt to be in optimal position, 1 cc of radio contrast dye is injected under continuous fluoroscopy. It is advisable to attach a low volume extension tubing to the needle, and inject the dye and subsequent medications via the extension tubing under continuous fluoroscopy. Care is taken to see that there is appropriate dye flow pattern, and it is critical to ensure that there is no intravascular dye spread. Continuous fluoroscopy is used because intravascular injection can be missed if intermittent fluoroscopy is used. In fact some people recommend routine use of digital subtraction to rule out intravascular injection, however this has not become a standard of care.

Once appropriate dye spread is confirmed, the steroid mixture can then be injected. Use of non-particulate steroid preparation is preferable because then there is less chance of vascular thrombosis.

When using this approach for the L5S1 interspace, it may require a caudal cranial adjustment of the C-arm to get appropriate visualization of the target by moving the superior articular process away.

The approach to the S1 foramen is different from the above. In this case the needle is placed through the posterior S1 foramen onto the pedicle of S1. The C-arm needs to be adjusted slightly cephalo-caudad and slightly ipsilateral oblique to superimpose the anterior and posterior S1 foramen. The needle enters at the lateral margin of the posterior S1 foramen. The safe technique is to initially hit the bony surface of the sacrum first, and then walk off into the foramen. At this point depth is checked in the lateral position to make sure the needle does not pass anteriorly into the pelvic cavity. Once needle is felt to be in appropriate position radiocontrast dye is injected to ensure appropriate dye spread along the S1 nerve root sleeve. At this point the mixture of cortisone is injected. Note that the dye and the subsequent medications should be injected under continuous fluoroscopy (Figs 25.2A to F and 25.3A to F).

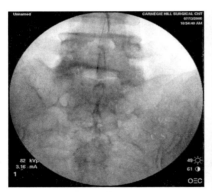

Fig. 25.2A: Straight AP view

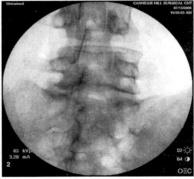

Fig. 25.2B: Slight oblique angulation with skin marker

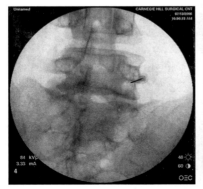

Fig. 25.2C: Needle entry-oblique view

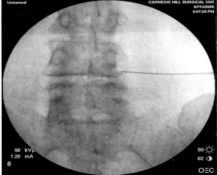

Fig. 25.2D: Reconfirm in AP view

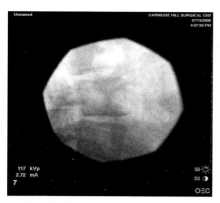

Fig. 25.2E: Lateral view of needle tip

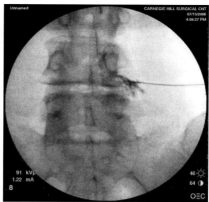

Fig. 25.2F: Final view of dye spread

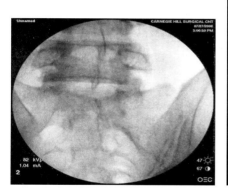

Fig. 25.3A: AP view

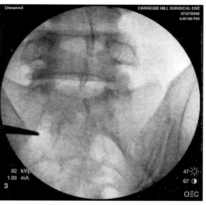

Fig. 25.3B: Needle entry point for S1

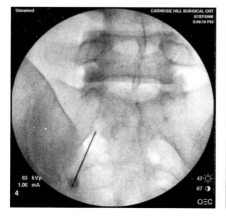

Fig. 25.3C: Needle headed towards
S1 foramen

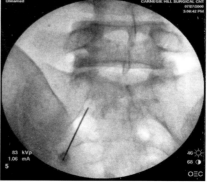

Fig. 25.3D: Needle walks off bone

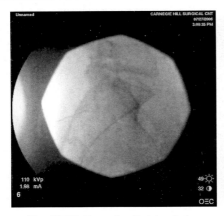

Fig. 25.3E: Reconfirm in lateral view

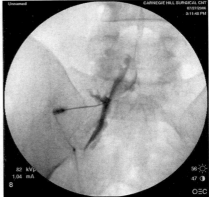

Fig. 25.3F: AP view of dye spread

Caudal Approach

After informed consent, patient is placed prone on the fluoroscopy table, with a pillow under the lower abdomen. Skin is prepped and draped in a sterile fashion. It is often helpful to have the patients rotate their feet inwards.

This procedure is ideally started with the C-arm in the lateral position. It is helpful usually to manually feel for the indentation of the sacral cornua. At this point skin and subcutaneous tissues are anesthetized.

Under lateral view of the fluoroscope, the needle is advanced cephalad towards the sacral hiatus at a 45 degree angle. If you touch bone, readjust the needle angle and try to walk the needle into the caudal canal. You will initially feel the needle entering the sacrococcygeal ligament, followed by the loss of resistance. At this point radiocontrast dye is injected and appropriate dye spread is reconfirmed in both lateral and AP positions. Careful negative aspiration is done before dye injection to ensure that no blood or CSF is aspirated.

Since the caudal canal is spacious, usually 10 to 15 cc of steroid mixture is injected (Figs 25.4A to E).

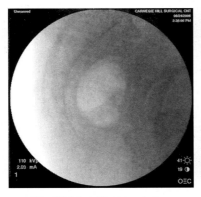

Fig. 25.4A: Initial lateral view

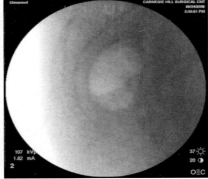

Fig. 25.4B: Needle headed towards canal

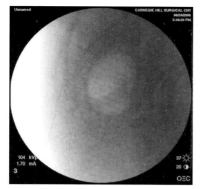

Fig. 25.4C: Needle walked into caudal canal

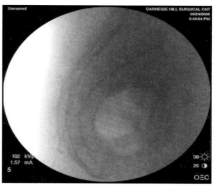

Fig. 25.4D: Dye spread in lateral view

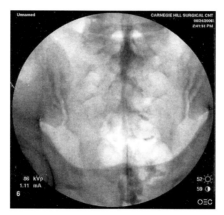

Fig. 25.4E: Dye spread in AP view

Post-procedural Care

Following the injection the patient should be monitored with physiological monitoring for at least 30 minutes. If vital signs are stable and the patient is doing well they may then be discharged. The patient should be advised of home care instructions including possible bruising and increased pain at the incision site for first few days following the procedure, in which ice packs may be beneficial, rest and abstinence from driving for 24 hours post procedure, increased activity as tolerated. The patient should rotify the office of any skin rashes, hives shortness of breath, wheezing, ii rease in pain level, persistent nausea or vomiting, persistent headache which worsens upon sitting, and fever greater than 100°F.

Complications

Potential risks are infrequent and divided into complications of needle placement or medication side effects. Possible risks of needle placement are pain at the injection site, nerve root injury, spinal cord injury, epidural hematoma, epidural abcess, meningitis, osteomyelitis, and postdural puncture headache. Local anesthetic side effects include weakness in lower extremity secondary to motor block, cardiac arrhythmia, seizure, and hypotension.[20] Patients should also be advised of potential steroid effects such as fluid retention, transient weight gain, hyperglycemia, hypertension, cushing syndrome, facial flushing, and steroid myopathy.[21] Allergic reactions may also occur with any of the medication administered.

Added precaution should be used when performing transforaminal epidural steroid injections. A case report[22] warned of 3 cases of unexpected paraplegia following lumbar transforaminal injections. The mechanism of injury was not demonstrated, but was referred to be inadvertent, intra-arterial injection of particulate steroids into a radicular artery that reinforced blood supply of the lower end of the spinal cord. This reinforces the need of careful attention when injecting the contrast medium to avoid possible intra-arterial injection of steroids.

CONCLUSION

Lumbar epidural steroid injections performed under fluoroscopic guidance are a safe and effective treatment modality for many conditions causing back pain and radicular symptoms. It should therefore be considered in the treatment plan in patients with a diagnosed, non-emergent cause of back pain who have failed more conservative treatment options.

REFERENCES

1. Derby R, Kine G, Saal J, Reynolds J, Goldthwaite N, White A, Hsu K, and Zucherman J. Response to steroid and duration of radicular pain as predictors of surgical outcome. Spine 1992;17:S176-83.
2. Derby R, Bogduk N, Kine G. Precision percutaneous blocking procedures for localizing spinal pain. Part 2. The lumbar neuraxial compartment. Pain Digest 1993; 3:175-88.
3. Bogduk N, Aprill C, Derby R. Epidural steroid injections. In: White AH (Ed), Spine Care, Volume One: Diagnosis and Conservative.
4. Bogduk N. Spine update: Epidural steroids. Spine 1995;20:845-8.
5. Dilke TFW, Burry HC, Grahame R. Extradural corticosteroid injection in the management of lumbar nerve root compression. BMJ 1973; 2:635-7.
6. Carrete S, Leclaire R, Marcoux S, et al. Epidural corticosteroid injections for sciatica due to herniated nucleus pulposus. N Engl J Med 1997; 336:1634-40.
7. Snoek W, Weber H, Jorgensen B. Double-blind evaluation of extradural methylprednisolone for herniated lumbar disc. Acta Orthop Scand 1977; 48:635-41.
8. Ridley MG, Kingsley GH, Gibson T, et al. Outpatient lumbar epidural corticosteroid injection in the management of sciatica. Br J Rheumatol 1988; 27:295-9.
9. Cuckler JM, Bernini PA, Wiesel SW, et al. The use of epidural steroids in the treatment of lumbar radicular pain. A prospective, randomized, double-blind study. J Bone Joint Surg Am 1985;67:63-6.

10. Bush K, Hillier S. A controlled study of caudal epidural steroid injections of triamcinolone plus procaine for the management of intractable sciatica. Spine 1991; 16:572-5.

11. Rapp SE, Haselkorn JK, Elam K, et al. Epidural steroid injection in the treatment of low back pain: A meta-analysis. Anesthesiology 1994; 81:A923.

12. Rydevik B, Brown MD, Lundborg G. Pathoanatomy and pathophysiology of nerve root compression. Spine 1984; 9:7-15.

13. Saal JS, Franson RC, Dobrow R, et al. High levels of inflammatory phospholipase A2 activity in lumbar disc herniations. Spine 1990;15:674-8.

15. Johansson A, Hao J, Sjolund B. Local corticosteroid blocks transmission in normal nocioceptive C-fibers. Acta Anesthesiol Scand 1990; 34:335-8.

16. Fuxe K, Harfstrand A, Agnati LF, et al. Immunocytochemical studies on the localization of glucocorticoid receptor immunoreactive nerve cells in the lower brain stem and spinal cord of the male rat using monoclonal antibody against rat liver glucocorticoid receptor. Neuroscience Lett 1985; 60:1-6.

17. Fenton DS, Czervionke LF. Image-Guided Spine Intervention. Saunders Philadelphia 2003; 100.

18. Bogduk N, Aprill C, Derby R. Selective nerve root blocks. In: Wilson DJ (Ed), Interventional radiology of the musculoskeletal system. Edward Arnold, London 1995;10:121-32.

19. Bogduk N, Aprill C, Derby R. Epidural steroid injections. In: White AH (Ed), Spine Care, Volume One: Diagnosis and conservative treatment. Mosby, St Louis 1995; 22:322-43.

21. Botwin KP, Gruber RD, Bouchlas CG, Torres-Ramos FM, Freeman TL, Slaten WK. Complications of fluoroscopically guided transforaminal lumbar epidural steroid injections. Arch Phys Med Rehabil 2000; 81:1045-50.

22. Houten JK, Errico TJ. Paraplegia after lumbosacral nerve root block: Report of three cases. The Spine Journal 2002; 2:70-75.

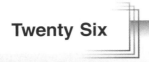

Twenty Six

Lumbar Facet and Median Branch Block

S Bakshi, GW Abrahamsen

INTRODUCTION

The facet joint is a true synovium-lined joint located in the posterior compartment of the spine that allows the spine to flex, extend, and rotate. The major causes of facet mediated back pain are osteoarthritis, erosions of the adjacent bone margins of the facets, bony overgrowth of the facets and articular processes, degenerative conditions resulting in reduction or loss of facet joint cartilage, or acute causes such as instability of the joint itself after trauma such as a motor vehicle accident. Facet pain is often an under diagnosed cause of back pain. However, the prevalence of facet joint mediated pain in patients with chronic spinal pain has been established as 15 to 40% of lower back pain.[1-3] Facet mediated pain is more common in the elderly than the younger population.

Facet mediated back pain has been studied for many years. Many studies have also been performed demonstrating facet mediated pain with the resolution of symptoms following injection of local anesthetic. In 1997 and 1998. Dreyfuss and colleagues, as well as, Kaplan et al performed studies demonstrating that lumbar medial branch blocks are target-specific and a valid test of zygapophysal joint pain.[4,5] Once the diagnosis has been established through lumbar medial branch blocks numerous studies have shown dramatic and long lasting relief of pain following lumbar medial branch neurotomy.[6,7]

Evaluation

Diagnosing facet mediated back pain should first begin with a detailed history and focused physical examination. One should suspect facet disease if the patient is complaining of poorly localized lower back pain that may be referred to the hip or thigh. These patients may also be employed in occupations that require repeated or excessive hyperflexion, hyperextension, or twisting movements of the spine. The physical examination may reveal facet tenderness and pain upon extension or lateral bending of the spine. Otherwise, the patient is neurologically intact. Referred pain to the lower extremities is not a contraindication for lumbar medial branch blocks. Pain referred as far as the leg and foot has been relieved by anesthetizing lumbar zygapophysial joints.[8,9]

Imaging studies are helpful but may be unreliable indicators of facetogenic pain.[10] Multiple studies have shown a lack of correlation between the results of conventional clinical examination and the response to controlled blocks.[11-14] This is the reason why a detailed history and examination in conjunction with facet joint injections and medial branch blocks play a vital role in the diagnosis and management of facetogenic pain.

ANATOMY

In order to accurately and completely diagnose and manage facet mediated pain, one must understand the anatomy of the spine. The spine can be broken up into three compartments: anterior, middle, and posterior. The anterior compartment consists of the vertebral bodies and disc spaces, the middle compartment consists of the epidural space and the neural foramina, and the posterior compartment consists of facet and sacroiliac joints. The zygapophysial joints (facet joints) are synovial joints between the superior and inferior articular processes of adjacent vertebrae. Each joint is surrounded by a thin, loose articular capsule. The capsule is attached to the margins of the articular processes of adjacent vertebrae. Accessory ligaments unite the laminae, transverse processes, and spinal processes and help stabilize the joint.[15]

The zygapophysial joints are innervated by articular branches that arise from the medial branches of the dorsal primary rami of the spinal nerves. As these nerves pass posteroinferiorly, they lie in groves on the posterior surfaces of the medial parts of the transverse processes. Each articular branch supplies two adjacent joints; therefore, each joint is supplied by two nerves. Thus, for example, the L3-4 joint is innervated by L2 and L3 medial branches. (Table 26.1)

Table 26.1: Innervation of various zygapophysial joints

Joint	Innervation
L2-3	L1, L2 MBB
L3-4	L2, L3 MBB
L4-5	L3, L4 MBB
L5-S1	L4, L5 MBB

Also keep in mind that the numbering of the medial branches differs from their location. Thus the L4 medial branch courses over the L5 transverse process and the L3 medial branch courses over the L4 transverse process.

Procedures

Once there is suspicion of facet mediated pain, the clinician then must decide to proceed with purely diagnostic medial branch blocks with local anesthetic or diagnostic and therapeutic intraarticular facet blocks with steroids. The clinician must also keep in mind that typically facet disease is not often limited to only one joint.

The purpose of performing medial branch blocks is to conclude if the patient's typical back pain is relieved by an injection of local anesthetic to the nerve. If the patient responds to the medial branch block, then a more permanent procedure, such as medial branch radiofrequency denervation can be considered. With this in mind, it is crucial to rule-out false-positive responses with the injection. Typically, 80% reduction of the patient's typical pre-procedure pain is considered a positive response. The clinician interpreting the results of the block must also consider placebo effect and the medial branch blocks are often repeated with a short-acting local anesthetic. A patient with 2 positive medial branch blocks concordant with the duration of action of the local anesthetic used should then be considered for medial branch rhizotomy.

Intra-articular facet blocks can also be considered for suspected facetogenic pain. This injection involves injecting a combination of a short or long-acting local anesthetic with a steroidal agent. This technique is thought to have a two-fold effect of diagnosing suspected facetogenic pain with the added benefit of reduction of inflammation from within the joint providing long lasting resolution of symptoms. However, it is felt that the longer lasting benefit of radiofrequency neurotomy after diagnosis with medial branch blocks is more beneficial then intra-articular injections with steroidal agents.

At this time the current guidelines of the International Spine Intervention Society state that lumbar medial branch blocks have replaced, or should replace, intra-articular injections in the diagnosis of lumbar zygapophysial joint pain, stating: Medial branch blocks are relatively easier to perform, medial branch blocks are safer and more expedient, medial branch blocks are more easily subjected to controls, intra-articular blocks lack therapeutic utility, i.e. if positive, they lack a valid subsequent treatment, medial branch blocks do have therapeutic utility for, if positive, the pain can be treated by radiofrequency neurotomy.[16]

CONTRAINDICATIONS

Absolute contraindications to medial branch and intra-articular injections include infection, anti-coagulation therapy, and pregnancy. If a patient is on anticoagulants medical clearance should be obtained from the treating physician to discontinue anticoagulants and a PT/PTT, INR should be obtained prior to the procedure. The clinician initiating these treatment modalities should also use caution if patient has known allergies to contrast dye and/or local anesthetics. Concurrent treatment with anti-inflammatory medication and aspirin should be stopped prior to the injections to prevent uncontrolled bleeding.

Equipment

These blocks are typically performed in a fluoroscopy suite under sterile technique using a C-arm fluoroscope. Equipment needed usually consists of sterile gloves and drapes, iodine based solution or alcohol-based antiseptic for skin preparation, 2 to 5 mm syringes, 25-gauge needle to anesthetize the skin, spinal needles 22 to 25-gauge 3.5 inch (1 per level), and a 18-gauge needle to draw up medication.

Medication

The typical local anesthetics used are bupivacaine 0.5% and lidocaine 2%. Omnipaque is used as the contrast medium. In addition, triamcinolone or depo medrol is used when performing intra-articular blocks. When performing medial blocks, no more than 0.5 ml is required to block the nerve adequately.

Techniques

Lumbar Facet Joint Injection

After informed consent is obtained, patient is placed on the fluoroscopy table with a pillow under the lower abdomen. Skin is prepped and draped in a sterile fashion.

Initial AP view of the spine is visualized. Once you reconfirm the exact level at which you want to perform the injection, the C-arm is rotated obliquely until the posterior part of the facet joint just begins to open. The angle will vary with the level of the joint being injected, since the upper lumbar facet joints have a different orientation than the lower lumbar facet joints. The ideal point of skin entry is just lateral to the inferior edge of the inferior articular process. Usually this is the widest part of the joint and is easiest to enter. This point is marked on the skin, and 1% lidocaine is used to anesthetize the skin and subcutaneous tissues.

At this point a 22 or 25-gauge spinal needle is used to enter the joint space using a "tunnel" approach. Often a pop is felt as you enter the joint space. This may or may not reproduce the patient's typical concordant pain. Injecting about 0.25 cc of radio contrast dye into the joint reconfirms appropriate position of the needle in the joint. Once appropriate placement of the needle in the joint has been confirmed, a mixture of local anesthetic and cortisone is injected into the joint (Figs 26.1A to E).

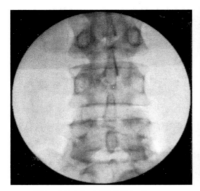

Fig. 26.1A: Initial AP view

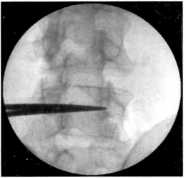

Fig. 26.1B: Oblique view with joint space opened up and marker on skin

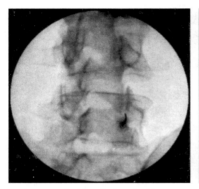

Fig. 26.1C: Needle headed into joint space

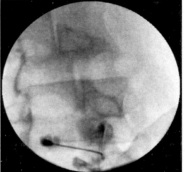

Fig. 26.1D: Dye spread within joint space AP view

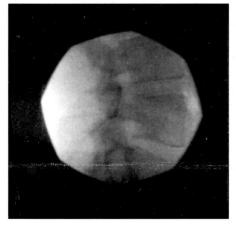

Fig. 26.1E: Lateral view of dye spread

Medial Branch Block

After informed consent is obtained, patient is placed on the fluoroscopy table in the prone position with a pillow placed under the lower abdomen. Skin is prepped and draped in a sterile fashion.

The procedure is started with a straight AP position of the C-arm. The C-arm is then rotated in an oblique fashion till the "Scotty dog" configuration is visualized. For the medial branches L1 to L4 the target position for the needle lies at the junction of the base of the transverse process and the superior articular process.

Under fluoroscopic guidance a 22 or 25-gauge spinal needle is advanced to this target position. Once the needle hits bone at this point, it is walked off the bone. Needle position is then checked in lateral position to make sure that it is not too far into the neural foramen.

At this point some people recommend injecting a small volume of radiocontrast dye to confirm that there is no vascular uptake. Once you have confirmed that needle is in the correct position, 0.3 to 0.5 cc of local anesthetic solution is injected to anesthetize the appropriate medial branch. It should be noted that the procedure for blocking the medial branch at L5 differs from the above procedure since the target point here is the superomedial aspect of the sacral ala. Once again, after the needle hits bone at this point, it should be walked off the bone slightly to ensure that the needle lies in contact with the nerve.

It is critical to ensure that the appropriate nerves are selected depending on which joint is being investigated. For example, if one wants to block the L4 -5 joint, the medial branches to be blocked will be the L3 and L4 nerves, which run at the level of the L4 and L5 transverse process respectively (Figs 26.2A to F).

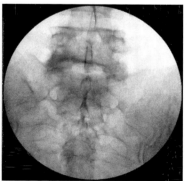 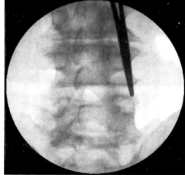

Fig. 26.2A: Initial AP view

Fig. 26.2B: Oblique view with marker on skin for L4 MBB block

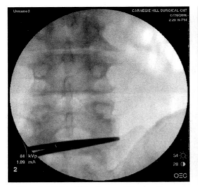

Fig. 26.2C: AP view with marker for L5 MBB Block

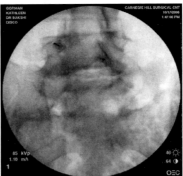

Fig. 26.2D: Needle at L4 MBB

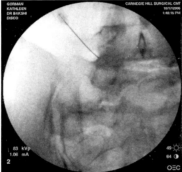

Fig. 26.2E: Needle at L5 MBB

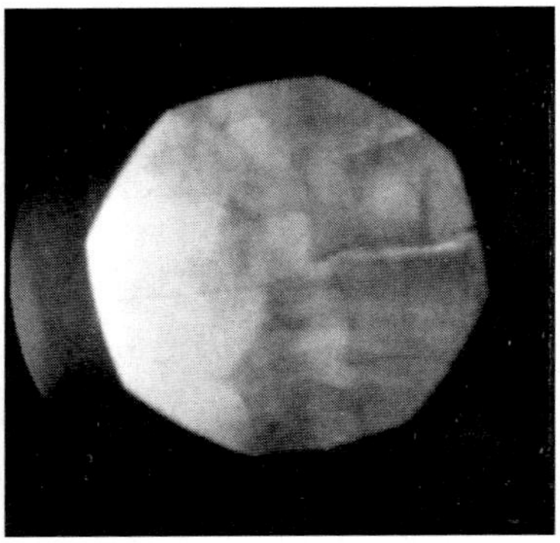

Fig. 26.2F: Lateral view of needle position

Post-procedural Care

The patient is discharged with postprocedural instructions to contact the office immediately in cases of increased temperature, onset of rash, new onset weakness in the extremities, severe unrelieved pain, etc. The patient should also be given a detailed explanation on how to accurately record their response to the injection and should follow-up in the office in 3 to 4 days. The patient can resume normal activities the following day and should refrain from driving or operating heavy machinery the day of the procedure. In cases where steroids are used, it may take 3 to 5 days for the full effect of the medication to take place.

Potential Complications

Medial branch blocks and intra-articular injections are relatively safe procedures. However, potential complications include, bleeding, infection, post-procedural radicular or back pain, thecal sac puncture and subsequent spinal headache, allergic reaction to medication, and possible vasovagal reaction.

CONCLUSION

Medial branch and intra-articular blocks are extremely useful procedures in the diagnosis and management of facet mediated back pain. With proper training they are relatively easy procedures and are excellent predictors to long-term outcome of treatment with radiofrequency denervation to the medial branches.

REFERENCES

1. Manchikanti L. Facet pain and the role of neural blockade in its management. Curr Rev Pain 1999;3:348-8.
2. Bogduk N. International spinal injection society guidelines for the performance of spinal injection procedures. Part 1: Zygapophyseal joint blocks. Din J Pain 1997;13:285-302.
3. Schwarzer AC, Aprill CN, Derby R, et al. Clinical features of patients with pain stemming from the zygapophysial joints. Is lumbar facet syndrome a clinical entity? Spine 1994; 19: 1132-7
4. Dreyfuss P, Schwarzer AC, Lau P, Bogduk N. Specificity of lumbar medial branch and L5 dorsal ramus blocks: A computed tomography study. Spine 1997; 22:895-902.
5. Kaplan M, Dreyfuss P, Halbrook B, Bogduk N. The ability of lumbar medial branch blocks to anesthetize the zygopophysial joint. Spine 1998; 23:1847-52.
6. Van Kleef M, Barendse GAM, Kessels A, Voets HM, Weber WEJ, de Lange S. Randomized trial of radiofrequency lumbar facet denervation for chronic low back pain. Spine 1999;24:1937-42.
7. Dreyfuss P, Halbrook B, Pauza K, Joshi A, McLarty J, Bogduk N. Efficacy and validity of radiofrequency neurotomy for chronic lumbar zygapophysial joint pain. Spine 2000; 25:1270-77.
8. McCall IW, Park WM, O'Brien JP. Induced pain referral from posterior elements in normal subjects. Spine 1979; 4:221-2.
9. Mooney V, Robertson J. The facet syndrome. Clin Orthop 1976; 115:149-56.
10. Schwarzer AC, Wang SC, O'Driscoll D, et al. The ability of computed tomography to identify a painful zygapophysial joint in patients with chronic low back pain. Spine 1995; 20:907-12.
11. Schwarzer AC, Aprill CN, Derby R, et al. Clinical features of patients with pain stemming from the zygapophysial joints. Is lumbar facet syndrome a clinical entity? Spine 1994; 19: 1132-7
12. Schwarzer AC, Wang S, Bogduk N, McNaught PJ, Laurent R. Prevalence and clinical features of lumbar zygapophysial joint pain: A study in an Australian population with chronic lower back pain. Ann Rheum Dis 1995; 54:100-106
13. Schwarzer AC, Derby R, Aprill CN, Fortin J, Kine G, Bogduk N. Pain from the lumbar zygapophysial joints: A test of two models. J Spinal Disord 1994; 7:331-6.
14. Revel M, Poiraudeau S, Auleley GR, Payan C, Denke A, Nguyen M, Chevrot A, Fermanian J. Capacity of the clinical picture to characterize low back pain relieved by facet joint anesthesia. Proposed criteria to identify patients with painful facet joints. Spine 1998; 23:1972-7.
15. Moore KL, Dalley AF, et al. Clinically oriented anatomy. 4th edition. Lippencott Williams and Wilkins 1999.
16. Bogduk N. Practice guidelines for spinal diagnostic and treatment procedures. International spine intervention society 2004; 47-8.

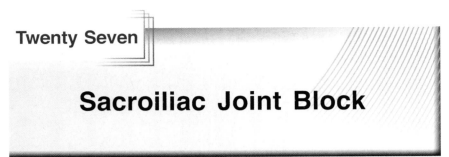

Twenty Seven

Sacroiliac Joint Block

S Gupta, J Richardson

INTRODUCTION

Intra-articular injection of local anesthetic into the sacroiliac joint (SIJ) is a diagnostic test that is used to confirm or refute that the pain is arising from the sacroiliac joint. If the pain is relieved it suggests that the targeted joint is the source of pain. However, injection of steroids into the SIJ can often provide satisfactory pain relief for several weeks or months allowing the patient to decrease oral medication.

Anatomy

The sacroiliac joint (SIJ) has a diffuse innervation, and the contributing nerves do not have a sufficiently fixed course such that they can all be selectively anesthetised and hence SIJ pain cannot be diagnosed using nerve blocks. A Japanese study of 18 cadavers, using macroscopic and histologic techniques, showed that the joint is innervated anteriorly from the ventral rami of L5 to S2 and via branches from the sacral plexus, and posteriorly from the lateral branches of the S1-4 dorsal rami.[1] The SIJ can be anesthetized only by intra-articular injections of local anesthetic.

Injections of corticosteroids into the sacroiliac joint have been shown to be efficacious in the treatment of sacroiliitis in some[2,3] but not all[4] controlled and observational, outcome studies. In clinical practice we see some patients respond with clinically significant pain relief for a significant duration which allows the patients to reduce the analgesic requirement with increased levels of activities.

Indications

The most important indication for SIJ blocks is to know if a patient's pain is arising from a SIJ or not. The risk of false-positive responses applies to all diagnostic blocks. One simple way of decreasing the incidence of false positive response is to repeat the block twice and if the patient gets good pain relief on two different occasions, the chances of a false positive response decreases. Establishing the diagnosis of SIJ pain may be worthwhile in order to prevent the patient pursuing futile investigations for other possible sources of pain.

History or physical examination may give us some idea if the pain may be arising for the SIJ but cannot accurately identify a painful SIJ. An area, about 3 x 10 cm in size, just inferior to the ipsilateral posterior superior iliac spine, is the characteristic site to which pain from the SIJ is referred in normal volunteers, referral to this area is common from other sources such as lumbar intervertebral disc and the lower lumbar facet joints. In patients with SIJ pain, the pain may be referred distally into the lower limb, but patterns of referral in the buttock, thigh, calf or foot do not distinguish SIJ pain from other sources of pain. Radiological studies including CT and MRI do not give any conclusive evidence if the pain is arising from the SIJ.

It has been established by several investigators that, in patients with SIJ pain, pain is always maximal below L5 [5-8]. Therefore, pain that is maximal above L5 is highly unlikely to be from the sacroiliac joint.

Contraindications

Absolute contraindications: Systemic or localized bacterial infection in the region of the block to be performed, bleeding diathesis, possible pregnancy.
Relative contraindications: Allergy to contrast medium or local anesthetic.

Equipment

Fluoroscopy is mandatory. The procedure is performed under aseptic conditions. 25G and 21G hypodermic needles, 2ml and 5 ml syringes are used.

A 22 or 25-gauge 100 mm spinal needle is commonly used. A slight curve at the distal 5 mm of the needle can be helpful to navigate the needle into the joint.

Intravenous solutions, sedation or antibiotics are not required.

Bupivacaine 0.5% or lignocaine 25% can be used with or without steroids (Methylprednosolone 40 mg or Triamcinolone 40 mg). Given the limited capacity of the sacroiliac joint about 2 to 3 ml is required to block the joint adequately.

Contrast medium is required to verify intra-articular placement of the needle.

Procedure

Baseline data concerning the location and extent of pain, including a pain score, and the movements and activities of daily living that are prevented by the pain are recorded so that these can be tested after the SIJ injection to establish if the pain is arising from the SIJ.

Informed consent must be obtained. Risk of infection, bleeding, and allergic reaction should be discussed.

The patient should lie prone on an operating table and the procedure is performed under aseptic conditions. Under AP view, the SI joint presents multiple sinuous lines running caudo-cranially, in a semi-parallel fashion (Fig. 27.1). As a rule, the more medial of these lines are formed by the posterior margins of the joint. In order to overlap the anterior and the posterior margins of the SIJ the C-arm should be rotated, usually to the contralateral side (as opposed to rotating the C-arm to ipsilateral side for facet joint block), so as to have all the margins superimposed along the caudal one-third of the joint line (Fig. 27.2). A target point is selected 1 to 2 cm cephalad of the inferior end of the joint line. After identifying the target point, local anesthetic is injected into the skin and subcutaneous tissue directly over the target point. A 22 or 25 g 100 mm curved tip needle is targeted to hit the sacrum (adding a slight bend to the distal 5 mm of the needle helps navigate the needle). Once the needle has struck the sacrum, it should be withdrawn slightly and redirected towards the joint space (Fig. 27.3). Entry into the joint can be recognized by loss of bony resistance as the tip slips between the sacrum and the ilium. On

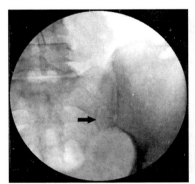

Fig. 27.1: AP view of the sacroiliac joint. The medial joint line is the posterior joint line (arrow)

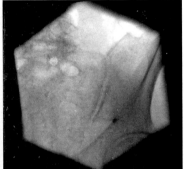

Fig. 27.2: The anterior and the posterior joint line have been superimposed by contralateral oblique rotation of the C-arm

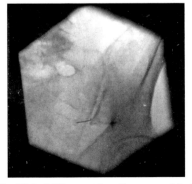

Fig. 27.3: A 22 g needle with a curved tip is seen entering the inferior part of the SI Joint

fluoroscopy, the tip will be seen to lie between the two bones. Sometimes, if not often, the tip of needle will be seen to bend slightly, as it wedges between the bones.

The tip of the needle should be inserted less than a few millimeters into the joint. If necessary, depth of insertion should be checked and evaluated on lateral imaging. Too great an insertion risks having the needle emerge from the anterior aspect of the joint into the presacral tissues. Arterial penetration can occur in this location.[4]

Once the needle has entered the joint space, intra-articular placement must be confirmed with an injection of contrast medium. If the needle has been correctly placed injection of 0.3 to 0.5 ml of contrast medium will outline the joint space. In postero-anterior views, the contrast medium should be seen to travel cephalad along the joint line (Fig. 27.4). In lateral views the contrast medium most densely outlines the perimeter of the joint (Fig. 27.5). Once correct intra-articular placement of the needle has been achieved 2.5 to 3.0 ml local anesthetic with or without steroid can be injected.

A different approach may be necessary if the above explained approach is unsuccessful or if the joint lines cannot be superimposed (Fig. 27.6). In order to isolate the posterior margin, the C-arm should be rotated, usually to the contralateral side, so as first to have all margins superimposed along the caudal one-third of the joint. Next, by rotating the C-arm in either direction, the anterior and posterior joint margins should be separated until they appear as separate entities. Rotation is then continued or adjusted until the cortical lines of the posterior joint is maximally crisp (Fig. 27.7). This orientation coincides with the beam being directed into the posterior opening of the inferior joint space. Usually, 5 to 20 degrees of contralateral rotation is necessary to properly image the inferior joint planes. A target point is selected 1 to 2 cm cephalad of the inferior end of the joint. This

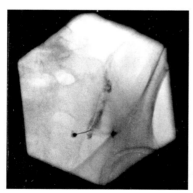

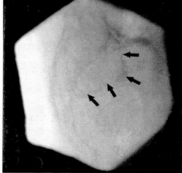

Fig. 27.4: Contrast medium spread along the SI joint (contralateral oblique view)

Fig. 27.5: Contrast medium spread can be seen along the perimeter of the joint line in lateral view as marked by the arrows

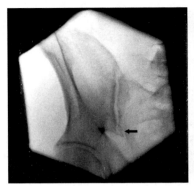 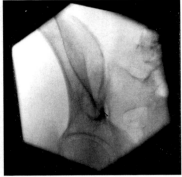

Fig. 27.6: The medial joint lines are the margins of the posterior SI joint line (arrow)

Fig. 27.7: With slight contralateral oblique rotation the posterior joint lines have become crisp and a curved tip needle is seen entering the joint

should be a zone of maximum radiolucency in the target region. A puncture point on the skin is selected directly overlying the target and the joint is entered as described above and contrast medium injected (Figs 27.8 and 27.9).

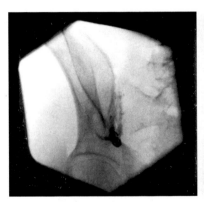 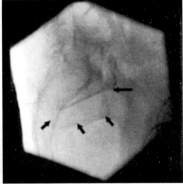

Fig. 27.8: Contrast medium spread along the SI joint line

Fig. 27.9: Lateral view showing the tip of the needle and the perimeter of the joint line as shown by the arrows

Post-procedural Care and Evaluation

After the injection, the patient should be monitored for 30 minutes to ensure that there is no lower extremity weakness or numbness resulting from leakage of local anesthetic onto the lumbosacral plexus via a ventral capsular tear or over penetration of the needle.

Appropriate discharge instructions should be given.

In clinical practice we observe that low back pain could be arising from more than one structure. One way of interpreting the block would be to assume that the degree of pain relief obtained is that which is arising from the SIJ in question. The International Spinal Intervention Society (ISIS) suggests that "it is prudent to consider a response negative if there is ≤ 50% pain relief, equivocal if there is 51 to 74% relief, and positive of there is at least 75% improvement, with the confidence that the response is truly positive as the percentage relief increases towards 100%. Moreover, any apparently positive response should be tested with a subsequent block to decrease the false positive response".[9]

Conclusion

SIJ pain is more common than we think. Studies have quoted the incidence of SIJ pain to be up to 15% among patients complaining of low back pain. If a patient has most of the pain below L5 level it is more likely to be arising from the SIJ. In our experience a mixture of local anesthetic and steroid can be useful in carefully selected patients who derive satisfactory pain relief for several weeks or months allowing them to reduce analgesic consumption with increased activities.

REFERENCES

1. Ikeda R. Innervation of the sacroiliac joint. Macroscopic and histologic studies. J Nippon Med School 1991;58:587-96.
2. Maugars Y, Mathis C, Berthelot J. Assessment of the efficacy of sacroiliac corticosteroid injection in spondylarthropathies. A double-blind study. Br J Rheum 1996;35:767-70.
3. Braun J, Bollow M, Seyrekbasan F, et al. CT Guided corticosteroid injection of the sacroiliac joint in patients with spondyloarthropathy with sacroiliitis. Clinical outcome and follow up by dynamic magnetic resonance imaging. J Rheumatol 1996;23:659-64.
4. Hanly JG, Mitchell M, MacMillan L, et al. Efficacy of sacroiliac corticosteroid injection in patients with inflammatory spondyloarthropathy: Result of a 6 month controlled study. J Rheumatol 2000;27:719-22.
5. Schwarzer AC, Aprill CN, Bogduk N. The sacroiliac joint in chronic low back pain. Spine 1995;20:31-7.
6. Maigne JY, Aivaliklis A, Pfefer F. Results of sacroiliac joint double block and value of sacroiliac pain provocation tests in 54 patients with low back pain. Spine 1996;21:1889-92.
7. Dreyfuss P, Michaelsen M, Pauza K, et al. The value of history and physical examination in diagnosing sacroiliac joint pain. Spine 1996; 21: 2594-2602.
8. Slipman C, Jackson H, Lipetz J, et al. Sacroiliac joint pain referral zones. Arch Phys Med Rehabil, 2000;81:334-8.
9. Sacroiliac Joint Block. In: Practice guidelines for spinal diagnosis and treatment procedures. N Bogduk (Ed). International Spine Intervention Society 2004: 66-85.

Section G

Advanced Pain
Management

Twenty Eight

Percutaneous Adhesiolysis for Failed Back Surgery Syndrome and Other Applications

Laxmaiah Manchikanti, Mark V Boswell,
Rinoo V Shah, James E Heavner

INTRODUCTION

The first reported epidural injection for chronic low back pain was performed in 1901.[1] The initial reports of epidurography were in 1921.[2] In ongoing efforts to manage chronic pain, cold hypertonic saline was administered intrathecally in 1967.[3] Subsequently, the use of intrathecal cold saline to relieve pain in cancer patients was reported.[4] The determining factor in the therapeutic effect of cold hypertonic solution was reported as its hypertonicity rather than the temperature.[5]

Racz et al[6,7] reported the first use of epidural hypertonic saline to facilitate lysis of adhesions and evaluated permeability of the dura in dogs in vitro, demonstrating slow transdural equilibration of hypertonic saline. Hyaluronidase was used in an attempt to alter the rapidity of onset and extent, intensity, and duration of caudal anesthesia.[8,9]

Over the years, multiple investigators[6,7,10-20] have studied the effectiveness of adhesiolysis and hypertonic saline neurolysis with or without hyaluronidase.

APPLIED ANATOMY

- The spine is divided anatomically into three compartments. These compartments have been defined as the anterior, neuroaxial, and posterior.[21]
  — The anterior compartment is comprised of the vertebral body and the intervertebral disc (Fig. 28.1).
  — The structures within the epidural space and neural pathways form the neuroaxial compartment, and the posterior compartment is composed of the posterior lamina and zygapophysial joints, along with the bony vertebral arch structures (Fig. 28.1).
- The anatomical orientation of the vertebral spinous processes are varied throughout the spinal axis.
  — In the lumbar spine, the spinous processes are directly above the widest portion of the interlaminar space, allowing both a midline and a paramedian approach to be relatively easy (Fig. 28.1).

- The neuraxial compartment consists of all structures within the osseous and ligamentous boundaries of the spinal canal (Fig. 28.1).
  — Within this compartment is the epidural space.
  — The epidural space contains fat, epidural veins, epidural arteries, and lymphatics.
  — The most common constituent of the epidural space is epidural fat.[22,23]
  — Epidural fat acts as a shock absorber to protect the contents of the epidural space and can also act as a depot for drugs and anesthetics injected into the epidural space.
- The spinal canal extends from the foramen magnum to the sacrum, which is bounded posteriorly by the ligamentum flavum and periosteum, anteriorly by the posterior longitudinal ligament that lies over the dorsal aspects of the vertebral bodies and discs and laterally by pedicles and intervertebral foramen.[24]
  — The spinal cord ends at L1 or L2 in adults and the dural sac continues to the spinal cord and conus, running down to the level of S2 (Fig. 28.1).[24]
- The dural sac rests on the floor of the vertebral canal.
- The anterior relations of the dural sac are the backs of the vertebral bodies and the intervertebral discs. Covering these structures is the posterior longitudinal ligament.
  — The anterior spinal arteries and sinuvertebral nerves run across the floor of the vertebral canal and are located anterior to the dural sac.
  — The dural sac posteriorly is related to the roof of the vertebral canal, the laminae, and ligamentum flava.
- The epidural space is a potential space intervening between the dural sac and the osseo-ligamentous boundaries of the vertebral canal (Fig. 28.1).
  — The epidural membrane is a thin layer of areolar connective tissue, which varies from diaphanous to pseudomembranous in structure.[24]
  — The epidural membrane surrounds the dural sac and lines the deep surface of the laminae and pedicles.
  — The epidural membrane lines the back of the vertebral body and then passes medially deep to the posterior longitudinal ligament, where it detaches to the anterior surface of the deep portion of the ligament, ventrally, opposite the vertebral bodies.
  — The posterior longitudinal ligament covers laterally the back of the disc, preventing the epidural membrane from covering the back of the annulus fibrosus.
  — The epidural space extends from the foramen magnum to the end of the dural sac at S2. The actual size of the posterior epidural space varies greatly. It expands to 4 to 6 mm at its greatest width in the mid-lumbar spine and gradually decreases to about 3 mm at the S1 level.
- The epidural space surrounds the dural sac.
  — It is bordered posteriorly by the ligamentum flavum and periosteum, and anteriorly by the posterior longitudinal ligament and vertebral bodies.
  — Laterally it is bordered by the pedicles and intervertebral foramina.

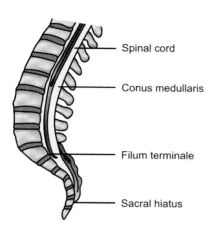

Spinal cord

Conus medullaris

Filum terminale

Sacral hiatus

A. Median sagittal section of the lumbosacral part of the vertebral column

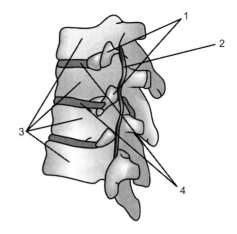

B. The ligamentum flavum
(1) Intervertebral foramen (2) Ligamentum flavum (3) Vertebral body (4) Intervertebral disc

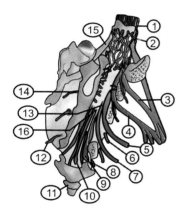

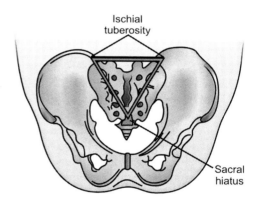

Ischial tuberosity

Sacral hiatus

C. Sacral canal, sacral nerves, and sacral venous plexus
(1) Dura Mater (2) Venous plexus (3) S1 anterior primary ramus (4) S2 nerve root (5) S3 nerve root (6) Posterior primary ramus (7) S4 nerve root (8) S5 nerve root (9) Coccygeal nerve (10) Filum Terminale (11) Coccyx (12) Posterior primary ramus (13) Termination of Dura Mater (14) 2nd posterior sacral foramen (15) L5 (16) Cauda equina

D. Identification of the sacral hiatus anatomical landmarks

Fig. 28.1: Anatomy of lumbosacral epidural space

— The epidural space is widest in the midline underneath the junction of the lamina and narrows laterally beneath the zygapophysial joint.
— Laterally the ligamentum flavum joins the joint capsule of the adjacent zygapophysial joint.
— The actual size and shape of the epidural space is determined by the manner of attachment of the dural sac to the walls of the spinal canal, as well as the shape of the spinal canal at different levels.
— Studies have demonstrated a dorsomedian connective tissue band in the lumbar epidural space. The posterior epidural space is divided by this dorsomedian connective tissue band (plica median dorsalis) and additional transverse connective tissue bands.
— However, controversy exists about whether the dorsomedian connective tissue is continuous, fenestrated or interrupted.
— The epidural space may be compartmentalized, which can account for the limitation of the injected substances.

- The ligamentum flavum has been proposed to be joined in the midline. There appears to be a paired nature to the ligament having both a right and left portion.
   — Cryomicrotome sectioning performed on the epidural space has shown that there is a variable degree of fusion of the ligamentum flavum in the midline.
   — The ligamentum flavum in the lumbar spine is thicker than in the cervical and thoracic spine.

- The sacrum is a triangular bone, dorsally convex, that consists of the five fused sacral vertebrae (Fig. 28.1). It articulates cephalad with the fifth lumbar vertebra and caudad with the coccyx.[21]
   — The concave anterior surface features four parts of large anterior sacral foramina that provide passage from the midline sacral canal for the anterior rami of the upper four sacral nerves.
   — The anterior foramina are unsealed and provide a ready escape passage for solutions injected into the sacral canal.
   — The dorsal surface of the sacrum is variably convex and irregular, with important prominences representing the fused elements of the sacral vertebrae.
   — In the midline, there is a median crest with three or more, but commonly four, prominent tubercles which are variable, representing the sacral spinous processes.[25] Lateral to the crest and medial to the four posterior sacral foramina is the intermediate sacral crest, with a row of four tubercles, which represent the upper four sacral articular processes (Fig. 28.1).
   — The remnants of the S5 inferior articular processes are prominent and palpable through the skin and constitute the sacral cornua and, together with adjacent coccygeal cornua which they abut, are key landmarks for identification of the sacral hiatus and successful caudal blockade.

- The coccyx is a small triangular bone consisting of three to five fused rudimentary vertebrae (Fig. 28.1).
  — The coccyx attaches to the lower part of the sacrum. The tip of the coccyx is an important landmark.
- The sacral hiatus is a defect in the lower part of the posterior wall of the sacrum, formed by the failure of laminae of S5, and usually part of S4, to meet and fuse in the median plane.
  — A variable space is left which is described as an inverted *U* or *V*, covered by the thick fibrous posterior sacral coccygeal ligament.[25]
  — Direct access to the caudal canal is obtained by penetration of the sacrococcygeal ligament.
  — There is significant variation in the normal anatomy in this area, with a widely and highly variable (in sizes and shapes) the sacral hiatus. The hiatus lies higher than the lower one-third of the S4 in about 50% of specimens.[25]
  — The distance between the tip of the dural sac and the apex of the hiatus is highly variable from 20 to 45 mm.
  — Absent hiatus has been described in approximately 7% of specimens, and very small (less than 2 mm) AP diameter of the canal at the apex of the hiatus in 5% of specimens. However, in practice, absent hiatus is probably seen in less than 1% of patients.

INDICATIONS AND CONTRAINDICATIONS

The purpose of percutaneous adhesiolysis is to eliminate the deleterious effects of scar formation, which can physically prevent direct application of drugs to nerves or other tissues to treat chronic back pain with or without radiculopathy, and to assure target delivery of drugs.

Indications are listed in Table 28.1.

Contraindications are listed in Table 28.2.

Adhesiolysis of epidural scar tissue, followed by the injection of

Table 28.1: Indications for lysis of epidural adhesions
• Duration of pain of at least 6 months
• Average pain levels of 5 on a scale of 0 to 10
• Intermittent or continuous pain causing functional disability
• Chronic low back and/or lower extremity pain which has failed to respond or poorly responded to non-interventional and non-surgical conservative management and fluoroscopically-directed epidural injections
• Chronic low back and/or lower extremity pain resulting from:
— Failed back surgery syndrome
— Epidural fibrosis
— Spinal stenosis
— Radiculopathy
— Small herniated discs
— Fractures of the vertebral bodies
— Vertebral metastases
— Degenerative diseases

Table 28.2: Contraindications for lysis of epidural adhesions

- Large contained or sequestered herniation
- Cauda equina syndrome
- Compressive radiculopathy
- Uncontrolled major depression or psychiatric disorders
- Uncontrolled or acute medical illnesses
- Chronic severe conditions that could interfere with the interpretations of the outcome assessments for pain and bodily function
- Pregnancy and lactation
- History of adverse reaction to local anesthetic, steroids, hypertonic saline or contrast
- Patients unable to understand the informed consent and protocol
- Patients unable to be positioned in prone position to perform the procedure
- Infection
- Anti-coagulant therapy
- Non-aspirin anti-platelet therapy

hypertonic saline, as described by Racz, Viesca, and others[6,7,19] involved on Day 1: epidurography, adhesiolysis, and injection of hyaluronidase, bupivacaine, triamcinolone diacetate, and 10% sodium chloride solution; injections of bupivacaine and hypertonic sodium chloride solution followed on days 2 and 3. Manchikanti et al[12-17] described and studied a modification of the Racz protocol modifying a 3 day procedure to a 1 day procedure.

Clinical effectiveness of percutaneous adhesiolysis was evaluated in three randomized, controlled trials,[11,16,17] and five retrospective evaluations,[6,12,14,15,18] with encouraging results.

Chopra et al[20], in a systematic review of the role of adhesiolysis in the management of chronic spinal pain, sought to answer multiple questions which included the following:

In managing chronic low back and lower extremity pain –
1. Is percutaneous adhesiolysis an effective treatment?
2. Is percutaneous adhesiolysis superior to epidural steroid injections?
3. Does the addition of hypertonic sodium chloride solution improve outcome?
4. Does the addition of hyaluronidase improve outcome?
5. Is percutaneous adhesiolysis a safe procedure?

The systematic review concluded that there was strong evidence to indicate effectiveness of percutaneous epidural adhesiolysis with administration of epidural steroids short-term and long-term in chronic, refractory low back pain and radicular pain. They also concluded that there was moderate evidence of effectiveness with the addition of hypertonic saline. They reported that the evidence of effectiveness of hyaluronidase was negative. They also concluded that adhesiolysis provided relief in patients who failed to respond with relief with epidural steroid injections. In addition, they also concluded that adhesiolysis with hypertonic saline neurolysis was a safe procedure with minimal complications when performed appropriately by trained hands. Results of published trials of percutaneous adhesiolysis and hypertonic saline neurolysis as utilized by Chopra et al[20] are listed in Table 28.3. In addition, evidence of adhesiolysis and hypertonic saline neurolysis analysis results are listed in Table 28.4.

TECHNICAL CONSIDERATIONS

The technique of lumbar adhesiolysis involves accessing the lumbar epidural space either by utilizing a caudal, interlaminar, or transforaminal approach. Entry is performed with a 16-gauge RK needle, followed by advancement of a Racz catheter into the epidural space, with appropriate lysis of adhesions under radiographic control utilizing nonionic contrast medium. Subsequently, a combination of local anesthetic and steroid is injected into the epidural space through the catheter; followed by hypertonic saline neurolysis which is carried out by a slow and intermittent injection of hypertonic saline, either by infusion or in incremental doses. In classic Racz technique, the procedure is repeated without steroids on Day 2 and Day 3; whereas, with other modifications, the catheter is removed after performing the initial procedure.

RACZ TECHNIQUE

The technique employed by Racz and colleagues,[6-11,19] is described as percutaneous epidural neuroplasty and is outlined in Table 28.5.

General Principles

- The consent form should include all possible complications related to the procedure.
- Intravenous access is strongly recommended.
  - It may be necessary to sedate the patient with midazolam and fentanyl. Although sedation is given, it is important that the patient be awake and responsive during the procedure to ensure that the spinal cord is not compressed during the injection.
- Fluoroscopy is mandatory.
- A water-soluble, nonionic contrast medium is used because of the possibility of unintended subarachnoid injection.

The Caudal Approach

- The patient is placed prone with a pillow under the abdomen to straighten the lumbar spine, with toes pointing inward.
- Monitors are applied, including electrocardiography sensors, a pulse oximeter, and a blood pressure cuff.
- The sacral area is prepared with sterile technique and draped from the top of the iliac crest to the bottom of the buttocks.
  - The sacral cornua and the sacral hiatus are palpated with the index finger of the operator's nondominant hand.

Table 28.3: Results of published trials of percutaneous adhesiolysis and hypertonic saline neurolysis

Study/Methods	Participants	Intervention(s)	Outcome(s)	Result(s)	Conclusion(s)
Manchikanti et al[17] A randomized, double blind trial	25 patients in Group I served as controls and were treated with catheterization but no adhesiolysis 25 patients in Group II were treated with catheterization, adhesiolysis, followed by injection of local anesthetic, normal saline, and steroid 25 patients in Group III consisted of adhesiolysis followed by injection of local anesthetic, hypertonic saline, and steroid	Experimental groups: Adhesiolysis, hypertonic saline neurolysis, steroid and local anesthetic and adhesiolysis, normal saline, steroid. Control group: Catheterization and no adhesiolysis	Timing: 3 months, 6 months, and 12 months Outcome measures: VAS pain scale, Oswestry Disability Index 2.0, Work status, opioid intake, range of motion measurements and psychological evaluation by P-3	72% of patients in Group III (adhesiolysis and hypertonic neurolysis), 60% of patients in Group II (adhesiolysis only), compared to 0% in Group I (control) showed significant improvement at 12-month follow-up	Positive short-term and long-term relief
Heavner et al[11] A randomized, double blind trial	59 patients with chronic intractable low back pain. All the patients failed conservative management, along with fluoroscopically directed epidural steroid injections.	Group I: hypertonic saline plus hyaluronidase Group II: hypertonic saline Group III: isotonic saline (0.9% NaCl) Group IV: isotonic saline plus hyaluronidase	Timing: 4 weeks, 3 months, 6 months. and 12 months Outcome measures: Pain relief	Initially 83% of the patients showed significant improvement compared to 49% of the patients at 3 months, 43% of the patients at 6 months, and 49% of the patients at 12 months	Positive short-term and long-term relief

Contd...

Contd...

Study/Methods	Participants	Intervention(s)	Outcome(s)	Result(s)	Conclusion(s)
Manchikanti et al[16] A randomized, controlled trial	45 patients were evaluated 15 patients in group I were treated conservatively 30 patients in group II were treated with percutaneous epidural adhesiolysis and hypertonic saline neurolysis	Experimental group: Adhesiolysis, hypertonic saline neurolysis and epidural steroid injection, one or more occasions. Control group: Physical therapy exercise program and medication	Timing: 1 month, 3 months, 6 months, 1 year Outcome measures: Pain relief, functional status, psychological status, employment status	Experimental group showed improvement with pain relief in 97% at 3 months, 93% at 6 months, and 47% of the patients at 1 year Generalized anxiety disorder, somatization disorder, average pain, and functional status improved significantly in Group II	Positive short-term and long-term relief
Manchikanti et al[14] A retrospective randomized evaluation	A retrospective randomized evaluation of the effectiveness of 1-day adhesiolysis and hypertonic saline neurolysis in 129 patients	Adhesiolysis, hypertonic saline neurolysis and injection of steroid	Timing: 4 weeks, 3 months, 6 months, 12 months Outcome measures: Pain relief	Initial relief was reported in 79% of the patients with 68% of the patients reporting relief at 3 months, 36% at 6 months and 13% at 12 months with 1 injection	Positive short-term and negative long-term relief

Contd...

Contd...

Study/Methods	Participants	Intervention(s)	Outcome(s)	Result(s)	Conclusion(s)
Manchikanti et al[15] A retrospective evaluation of 60 post lumbar laminectomy patients with chronic low back pain	60 post lumbar laminectomy patients were included after failure of conservative management	Adhesiolysis, hypertonic saline neurolysis and injection of steroid	Timing: 3 months, 6 months, 12 months Outcome measures: Pain relief	With multiple injections, initial relief was seen in 100% of the patients, however it declined to 90% at 3 months, 72% at 6 months, and 52% at 1 year	Positive short-term relief and long-term relief

Reproduced from Chopra et al.[20] Role of adhesiolysis in the management of chronic spinal pain: A systematic review of effectiveness and complications. *Pain Physician* 2005; 8:87-100 with permission from authors and American Society of Interventional Pain Physicians.

Table 28.4: Results of published reports of percutaneous lysis of lumbar epidural adhesions and hypertonic saline neurolysis

Study	Study Characteristics	Methodological Quality Score(s)		No. of Patients	Initial Relief	Long-term Relief			Results	
		AHRQ Score(s)	Cochrane Score(s)		< 3 months	3 months	6 months	12 months	Short-term < 3 months	Long-term > 3 months
Manchikanti et al[17]	RA, DB	10/10	10/10	G1=25 G2=25 G3=25	33% 64% 72%	0% 64% 72%	0% 60% 72%	0% 60% 72%	P	P
Heavner et al[11]	RA, DB	7/10	7/10	59	83%	49%	43%	49%	P	P
Manchikanti et al[16]	RA	5/10	6/10	C=15 Tx=30	NSI 97%	NSI 97%	NSI 93%	NSI 47%	P	P
Manchikanti et al[14]	R	4/8	---	129	79%	68%	36%	13%	P	N
Manchikanti et al[15]	R	4/8	---	60	100%	90%	72%	52%	P	P

RA = randomized; DB = double blind; R = retrospective; NA = not available; NSI - no significant improvement; P = positive; N = negative

Reproduced from Boswell et al[10] Interventional techniques in the management of chronic spinal pain: Evidence-based practice guidelines. *Pain Physician* 2005; 8:1-47 with permission from authors and American Society of Interventional Pain Physicians.

Table 28.5: Percutaneous epidural neuroplasty technique as per Racz and colleagues

In the operating room:
1. Place epidural needle.
2. Inject iohexol (omnipaque-240) and visualize spread of contrast medium (epidurogram).
3. If filling defect corresponding to area of pain is present, thread Racz Tun-L-Kath® (Epimed) catheter into filling defect (scar), while injected normal saline through the catheter; observe fluoroscopically to visualize washout of contrast and opening of scar.
4. Inject additional iohexol to ascertain opening of scar and spread of injectate within the epidural space.
5. Inject preservative-free saline with or without hyaluronidase (Wydase).
6. Inject 0.25% bupivacaine or 0.2% ropivacaine plus corticosteroid (4 mg dexamethasone or 40 mg methylprednisolone or triamcinolone).
7. Tape catheter in place.

In the postoperative care unit:
• Inject 0.9% or 10% saline 30 minutes after steroid/local anesthetic injection.

In clinic area:
1. Once on each of the following 2 days, inject 0.25% bupivacaine or 0.2% ropivacaine; 30 minutes later, inject 0.9% or 10% saline.
2. After the last treatment, remove the epidural catheter.

Adapted and updated from Heavner JE, et al.[11] Percutaneous epidural neuroplasty. Prospective evaluation of 0.9% NaCl versus 10% NaCl with or without hyaluronidase. *Reg Anesth Pain Med* 1999; 24:202-207 with permission from authors and American Society of Interventional Pain Physicians.

— The entry point through the skin, approximately 1 to 2 cm lateral and 2 cm inferior to the sacral hiatus, is in the gluteal fold opposite the affected side.
— The entry point is infiltrated with a local anesthetic such as lidocaine.
— A 16-gauge RK needle® is passed through the described entry point.
— The needle is advanced to a point below the S3 foramen to prevent S3 nerve root damage.
• Placement is confirmed by lateral and anteroposterior fluoroscopic views.
— After aspiration is negative for blood and cerebrospinal fluid (CSF), 10 mL of iohexol (Omnipaque®-240) or metrizamide (Amipaque®) is injected under fluoroscopy.
• Next, insert a catheter into the scarred area.
— The ideal epidural catheter is a stainless steel, fluoropolymer-coated, spiral-tipped Racz Tun-L-Kath-XL®(Epimed International Inc.) as illustrated in Fig. 28.2.
— The bevel of the needle should face the ventrolateral aspect of the caudal canal on the affected side.
— Multiple passes may be necessary to place the catheter into the scarred area.
— To facilitate steering of the catheter into the desired location, a 15 degree bend is placed at its distal end.

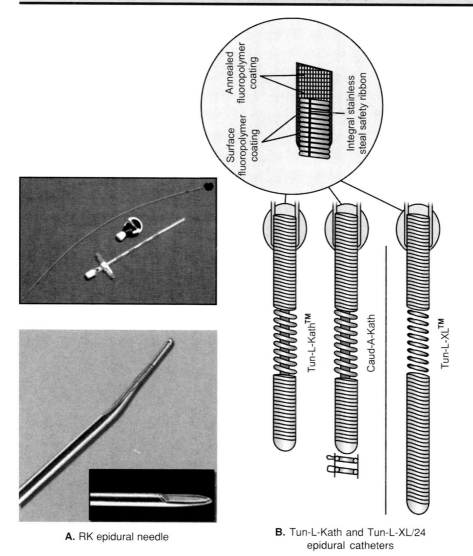

A. RK epidural needle

B. Tun-L-Kath and Tun-L-XL/24 epidural catheters

Fig. 28.2: Special needle and catheter for adhesiolysis
(Courtesy: Epimed International, Gloversville, NY, with permission)

- After final placement of the catheter and negative aspiration, another 5 to 10 mL of contrast medium is injected through the catheter
  — This additional contrast should spread into the area of previous filling defect and outline the targeted nerve root (Figs 28.3A to E). Fifteen hundred units of hyaluronidase (Wydase®) in 10 mL of preservative-free saline is injected rapidly.
  — Afterward, 10 mL of 0.2% ropivacaine or 0.25% bupivacaine and 40 mg of triamcinolone or methylprednisolone are injected through the catheter in divided doses. Other corticosteroids may also be used.

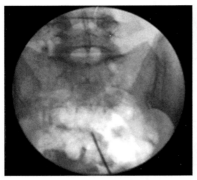

A. AP view of RK needle in place through the sacral hiatus

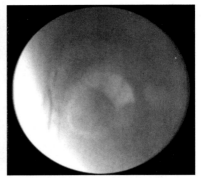

B. Lateral view with RK needle in place at sacral epidural space

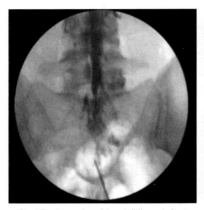

C. AP view of epidural filling defect

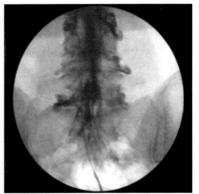

D. Catheter guided to lumbar epidural space (AP view)

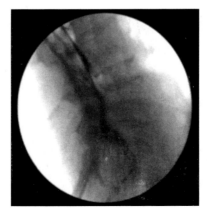

E. Lateral view of epidural filling

Fig. 28.3A to E: Caudal epidural adhesiolysis

- When the procedure is completed, the catheter should be secured to the skin with 2-0 nylon on a cutting needle, with application of antibiotic ointment and gauze.
  — The catheter is connected to an adapter and to a bacteriostatic filter that is not removed until three daily injections have been completed. The filter is capped, and the catheter is taped to the flank of the patient.
- During the procedure, the patient is given I.V. antibiotics in the form of cephalosporins (Rocephin®), 1g/day, to prevent bacterial colonization that is especially hazardous because of the epidurally-administered steroid.
- Once the patient is taken to the recovery room (placed with the affected side down) and vital signs are checked, 9 mL of 10% hypertonic saline is infused over 20 to 30 minutes.
  — Occasionally, the patient may complain of severe, burning pain during the infusion. The cause is usually the introduction of hypertonic saline into non-anesthetized epidural tissue.
  — Should the patient complain of pain, the infusion must be stopped and another 3 to 5 mL bolus of local anesthetic is given. After 5 minutes, the hypertonic saline infusion can be restarted without incident.
  — After completion of the hypertonic saline infusion, 1.5 mL of preservative-free normal saline is used to flush the catheter. Once this task is completed, the cap is replaced on the filter.
- The catheter is left in place for 3 days.
  — On the second and third days, it is injected once a day with 10 mL of 0.2% ropivacaine after negative aspiration from the catheter. Fifteen minutes later, 10 mL of 10% saline is infused over 20 minutes for patient comfort.
  — As in any hypertonic saline infusion series, the catheter must be flushed with 1.5 mL of preservative-free normal saline.
  — On the third day, the catheter is removed 10 minutes after the last injection.
  — A triple antibiotic ointment is placed on the wound, which is covered with a bandage or other appropriate dressing.

Interlaminar Lumbar Approach

The technique for lysis of epidural adhesions in these areas of the spinal cord must be modified to ensure that initially the needle is positioned in the epidural space and that spinal cord compression by subsequent injections is avoided.

- The patient is placed in the lateral or prone position on the fluoroscopy table.

— Sterile preparation and draping is carried out.
— Skin entry should be 1.5 to 2 levels below the desired epidural entry to facilitate catheter placement.

- After local anesthetic is used on the skin, an 18-gauge needle is inserted through the same puncture site to form an entry wound.
  — Through the puncture site, a 16-gauge RK needle is first advanced under fluoroscopic guidance (AP view) to determine the *direction* of the needle.
  — Next, in the lateral view, the needle is advanced to the point just before the "straight line" formed by the fluoroscopic image of the anterior border of the spinous process in the lateral view (the insertion site of the ligamentum flavum).
  — The lateral view under fluoroscopy demonstrates the *depth* of needle placement.
  — Lastly, an AP view is checked again to confirm the *direction* of the needle.
  — When the direction is satisfactory, the loss-of-resistance technique is used to advance the needle into the epidural space.
- Inject contrast to outline the filling defect.
- A Racz Tun-L-Kath or Racz Tun-L-Kath-XL epidural catheter is passed in an anterocephalad direction toward the filling defect outlined by the contrast, until the catheter tip enters the scarred area.
  — After negative aspiration, 1 to 3 mL of nonionic contrast is injected while observing the fluoroscope screen for spread within the adhesions and runoff of contrast is observed.
  — Once an outflow or runoff tract is seen (i.e. either opening of the neuroforamina or caudal spread), 3 to 5 mL of 0.9% preservative-free saline with 1500 units hyaluronidase is injected.
  — Lastly, 0.2% ropivacaine (4 mL) and 40 mg (1 mL) triamcinolone diacetate are injected after negative aspiration, while attention is directed to watch for displacement of the contrast.
  — For safety purposes, the local anesthetic is given in divided doses to first rule out intrathecal subdural (1-2 mL), or intravascular injection. Five minutes later the rest of the volume of the local anesthetic and steroid is injected.

MODIFIED MANCHIKANTI TECHNIQUE

The technique utilized by Manchikanti et al[16] is outlined in Table 28.6 and illustrated in Figs 28.4 to 28.6.

Facilities

The procedure is performed in a sterile operating room under appropriate sterile precautions utilizing fluoroscopy, RK needle, and a spring-wire catheter.

Table 28.6: Percutaneous epidural adhesiolysis technique

In the operating room:
1. Place epidural needle.
2. Inject omnipaque 240 and visualize spread of contrast medium with caudal or lumbar epidurogram.
3. After identification of the filling defect corresponding to the area of the pain, thread a Racz catheter into filling defect.
4. Inject additional omnipaque 240 to ascertain opening of the scar and spread of injectate within the epidural space and nerve roots.
5. Inject preservative-free saline 10-20 mL.
6. Inject 2% xylocaine 5 mL.
7. Tape the catheter in place in a sterile fashion.

In the recovery room:
1. After ascertaining for motor blockade, inject 6 mL of 10% saline in two divided doses of 3 mL each,
   15-30 minutes after injection of local anesthetic.
2. Inject 6-12 mg of celestone soluspan, or 40-80 mg of alcohol-free depo medrol, or 40-80 mg of triamcinolone.
3. Inject 0.5-1 mL of normal saline and remove the catheter.

Adapted and modified from Manchikanti et al.[16] Role of one day epidural adhesiolysis in management of chronic low back pain: A randomized clinical trial. Pain Physician 2001; 4:153-166 with permission from authors and American Society of Interventional Pain Physicians.

Preparation

After the initial evaluation, the patient is transferred to the holding area, where appropriate preparation is carried out, including preoperative evaluation, with I.V. access, and administration of antibiotic, based on protocol and patient condition.

Consent

An appropriate detailed consent is obtained from all patients.

Operating Room

- Procedural steps are illustrated in Figures 28.4A to D and 28.5A to F.
  - Patient is positioned in prone position.
  - Sterile preparation is carried out with povidone-iodine (Betadine®) prep.
  - Draping is carried out to cover the patient, extending into the midthoracic or cervical region.
  - Appropriate monitoring, of BP, pulse, and pulse oximetry is carried out.
  - Sedation is slowly administered.
  - The fluoroscope is adjusted over the lumbosacral region for AP and lateral views.

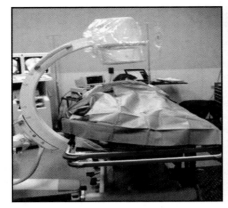

A. C-arm positioning in AP
position

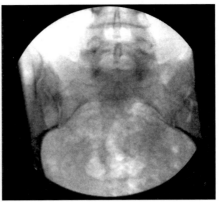

B. Fluoroscopic view in AP
position

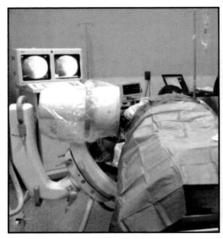

C. C-arm positioning in lateral position

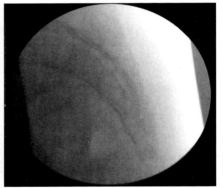

D. Fluoroscopic view in lateral position

Fig. 28.4A to D: Percutaneous adhesiolysis with caudal approach–positioning,
preparation and fluoroscopy

— A physician, scrubbed and in sterile gown and gloves, infiltrates the
area for needle insertion with local anesthetic.
— An RK needle is introduced into the epidural space under fluoroscopic utilization.
— Once the needle placement is confirmed to be in the epidural space, a
lumbar epidurogram is carried out utilizing approximately 2 to 5 mL
of contrast. Finding the filling defects by examining the contrast flow
into the nerve roots is the purpose of the epidurogram.
• After appropriate determination of epidurography, a Racz catheter, which
is a spring-guided, reinforced catheter, is slowly passed through the RK

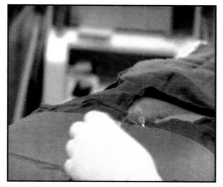

A. Catheter placement and adhesiolysis

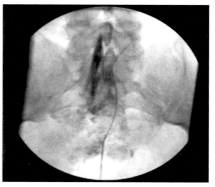

B. Fluoroscopic view of catheter placement

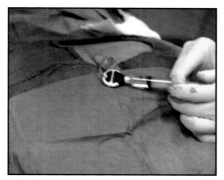

C. Contrast injection after adhesiolysis

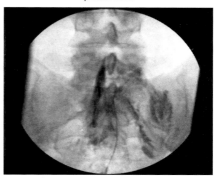

D. AP fluoroscopic view with filling of L5 and S1 nerve roots

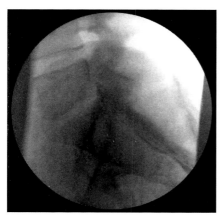

E. Lateral fluoroscopic view after completion

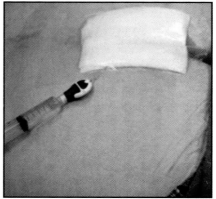

F. Appropriate dressing applied

Fig. 28.5A to F: Percutaneous adhesiolysis with caudal approach – catheter placement, adhesiolysis and epidurography

needle to the area of the filling defect or the site of pathology determined by MRI, CT, or patient symptoms.

— Following the positioning of the catheter into the appropriate area by mechanical means, adhesiolysis is carried out.

— After completion of the adhesiolysis, a repeat epidurogram is carried out by additional injection of contrast.

— If appropriate adhesiolysis is completed, nerve root filling as well as epidural filling will be noted. Figures 28.6A to F illustrates an example of the procedure.

— Figures 28.7A to C illustrates subarachnoid injection of contrast.

• At this time, variable doses of local anesthetic are injected. Commonly injected are 5 to 10 mL of 2% lidocaine hydrochloride or 5 to 10 mL of 0.25% bupivacaine.

• Following completion of the injection, the catheter is taped utilizing bio-occlusive dressing; and the patient is turned to the supine position and transferred to the recovery room.

Recovery Room

• The patient is very closely monitored for any potential complications or side effects. If no complications are observed and the patient reports good pain relief without any motor weakness, hypertonic saline neurolysis is carried out at this time by injection of variable doses of 10% sodium chloride solution.

— Hypertonic neurolysis may be carried out by an infusion pump or repeat injections in doses of 2 to 3 mL, ranging from 6 to 10 mL total, followed by injection of steroid (Celestone® 6 to 12 mg or Depo Medrol® 40 to 80 mg).[40]

• The catheter is flushed with normal saline, removed, and checked for intactness.

— The wound is also checked at this time.

• The patient is ambulated if all parameters are satisfactory. I.V. access is removed, and the patient is discharged home with appropriate instructions.

SIDE EFFECTS AND COMPLICATIONS

The most common and worrisome complications of adhesiolysis in the lumbar spine are related to dural puncture, spinal cord compression, catheter shearing, infection, steroids, hypertonic saline, and hyaluronidase.[19,20,26-38] Complications are listed in Table 28.7. Unintended subarachnoid or subdural puncture with injection of local anesthetic or hypertonic saline is one of the major complications of the procedure. Hypertonic saline injected into the subarachnoid space has been reported to cause cardiac arrhythmias, myelopathy, paralysis, and loss of sphincter control.[30] In fact, Aldrete et al[31] attributed incidences of arachnoiditis following epidural adhesiolysis with hypertonic saline to subarachnoid leakage of hypertonic saline. However, a

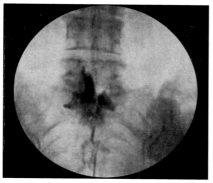

A. AP view of lumbar epidurogram

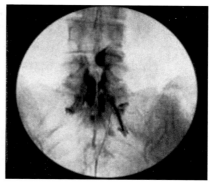

B. AP view contrast injection with right S1 nerve root filling

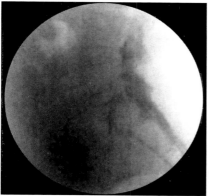

C. Lateral view of "C" with filling defect on right side

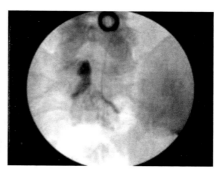

D. AP view showing defect on right with Racz catheter in place

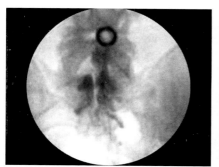

E. AP view following appropriate adhesiolysis

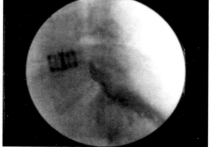

F. Lateral view of 'B'

Fig. 28.6A to F: Examples of caudal epidural adhesiolysis with right S1 radiculitis

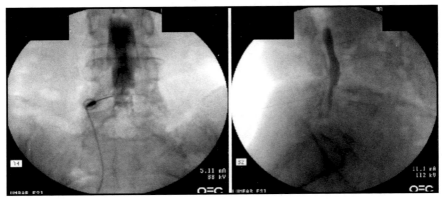

A. Lumbar interlaminar epidural with subarachnoid filling patterns – AP and lateral views

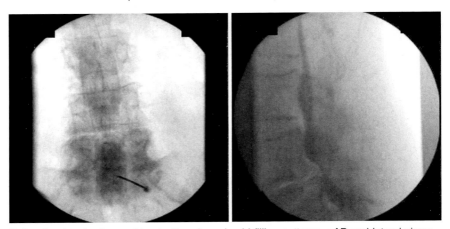

B. Lumbar interlaminar epidural with subarachnoid filling patterns – AP and lateral views

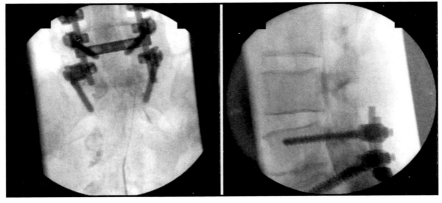

C. Caudal epidural adhesiolysis–subarachnoid distribution of contrast–AP and lateral views

Fig. 28.7A to C: Subarachnoid pattern of contrast injection

Table 28.7: Potential complications of percutaneous adhesiolysis

Pain
- Pain at the site of the needle insertion
- Exacerbation of existing pain
- Pain in the low back

Infection
- Soft tissue abscess
- Epidural abscess
- Meningitis
- Encephalitis

Bleeding
- Soft tissue hematoma
- Epidural hematoma
- Spinal cord hematoma
- Neve root sheath hematoma

Trauma
- Soft tissue
- Nerve root
- Spinal cord

Inadvertent injection
- Dural puncture
- Subdural injection
- Intrathecal injection
- Intravascular injection

Miscellaneous
- Spinal cord compression
- Cauda equina syndrome
- Arachnoiditis
- Paraplegia
- Increased intrathecal pressure
- Increased intraocular pressure
- Retinal hemorrhage
- Torn catheter
- Retained catheter

Local anesthetic effects
Steroid side effects

study of 108 patients suffering from intractable pain treated by intrathecal hypertonic saline, reported that sphincter disorders were present in 8% of the patients, with 2.7% experiencing cauda equina syndromes with paraplegia.[33] The study also reported rapid recovery in one patient, but quite slow and incomplete recovery in the others, attributing the cauda equina syndromes to pre-existing arachnoiditis in one patient and two arteriovascular diseases in the others. In a survey of 648 neurosurgeons and 1,943 patients treated for pain, it was reported that 31.2% had used intrathecal hypertonic saline with adverse reactions in 11.2% of the patients as compared to adverse reactions in only 7.6% of those treated with normal or diluted saline injections.[34] Twenty-two patients, or 1%, suffered significant morbidity with paraplegia or tetraplegia in 16, or 0.76% of the patients, and monoparesis in one patient (0.05%).

The second specific complication of percutaneous epidural adhesiolysis is related to catheter shearing and its retention in the epidural space. Even though the RK needle (Epimed International Inc.) and Racz Catheter (Epimed International Inc.) have been specifically designed for this procedure, catheter shearing has been reported. Racz et al[19] reported this problem as occurring in five such cases. Manchikanti and Bakhit[32] also reported a torn Racz catheter in the lumbar epidural space, which was successfully removed. Spinal cord compression following rapid injections into the epidural space, epidural infection, direct trauma to the spinal cord, neural trauma, and occasional sensitivity (3%) to hyaluronidase are potential complications.[36-38] Other side effects are related to the administration of steroids and are generally attributed to the chemistry or pharmacology of the steroids.[26] However, therapeutic doses of epidural steroids in appropriate dosing was without complications.[39]

REFERENCES

1. Sicard MA. Les injections medicamenteuse extraduraqles per voie saracoccygiene. Comptes Renues des Senances de la Societe de Biolgie et de ses Filliales 1901;53:396-8.
2. Sicard JA, Forestier J. Methode radiographique d'exploration de la cavite epidurale par le Lipiodol. Rev Neurol 1921;2:1264.
3. Hitchcock E. Hypothermic subarachnoid irrigation for intractable pain. Lancet 1967;1:1133-5.
4. Ventrafridda V, Spreafico R. Subarachnoid saline perfusion. In Bonica JJ (Ed.), Advances in Neurology, Vol. 4. Raven Press, New York, 1974, 477-84.
5. Hitchcock E. Osmolytic neurolysis for intractable facial pain. Lancet 1969;1:434-6.
6. Racz GB, Holubec JT. Lysis of adhesions in the epidural space. In Racz GB (Ed.), Techniques of Neurolysis. Kluwer Academic Publishers, Boston, 1989;57-72.
7. Racz GB, Heavner JE, Singleton W, Caroline M. Hypertonic saline and corticosteroid injected epidurally for pain control. In Raj P (Ed), Techniques of Neurolysis. Kluwer Academic Publishers, Boston, 1989;73-86.
8. Payne JN, Rupp NH. The use of hyaluronidase in caudal block anesthesia. Anesthesiology 1951;2:161-72.
9. Moore DC. The use of hyaluronidase in local and nerve block analgesia other than spinal block. 1520 cases. Anesthesiology 1951;12:611-26.
10. Boswell MV, Shah RV, Everett CR, Sehgal N, McKenzie-Brown AM, Abdi S, Bowman RC, Deer TR, Datta S, Colson JD, Spillane WF, Smith HS, Lucas-Levin LF, Burton AW, Chopra P, Staats PS, Wasserman RA, Manchikanti L. Interventional techniques in the management of chronic spinal pain: Evidence-based practice guidelines. Pain Physician 2005;8:1-47.
11. Heavner JE, Racz GB, Raj PP. Percutaneous epidural neuroplasty. Prospective evaluation of 0.9 percent NaCl versus 10 percent NaCl with or without hyaluronidase. Reg Anesth Pain Med 1999;24:202-7.
12. Manchikanti L, Pampati VS, Rivera JJ, Fellows B, Beyer CD, Damron KS, Cash KA. Effectiveness of percutaneous adhesiolysis and hypertonic saline neurolysis in refractory spinal stenosis. Pain Physician 2001;4:366-73.
13. Manchikanti L, Bakhit CE. Percutaneous lysis of epidural adhesions. Pain Physician 2000;3:46-64.

14. Manchikanti L, Pakanati RR, Bakhit CE, Pampati VS. Role of adhesiolysis and hypertonic saline neurolysis in management of low back pain. Evaluation of modification of Racz protocol. Pain Digest 1999;9:91-6.

15. Manchikanti L, Pampati VS, Bakhit CE, Pakanati RR. Non-endoscopic and endoscopic adhesiolysis in post lumbar laminectomy syndrome. A one-year outcome study and cost effectiveness analysis. Pain Physician 1999; 2:52-8.

16. Manchikanti L, Pampati VS, Fellows B, Rivera JJ, Beyer CD, Damron KS. Role of one day epidural adhesiolysis in management of chronic low back pain: A randomized clinical trial. Pain Physician 2001;4:153-66.

17. Manchikanti L, Rivera JJ, Pampati VS, Damron KS, McManus CD, Brandon DE, Wilson SR. One day lumbar epidural adhesiolysis and hypertonic saline neurolysis in treatment of chronic low back pain: A randomized, double-blind trial. Pain Physician 2004;7:177-86.

18. Hammer M, Doleys D, Chung O. Transforaminal ventral epidural adhesiolysis. Pain Physician 2001;4:273-9.

19. Viesca CO, Racz GB, Day MR. Special techniques in pain management: Lysis of adhesions. Anesthesiol Clin North Am 2003;21:745-66.

20. Chopra P, Smith HS, Deer TR, Bowman RC. Role of adhesiolysis in the management of chronic spinal pain: A systematic review of effectiveness and complications. Pain Physician 2005;8:87-100.

21. Kuslich SD, Ulstrom CL, Michael CJ. The tissue origin of low back pain and sciatica: A report of pain response to tissue stimulation during operation on the lumbar spine using local anesthesia. Orthop Clin North Am 1991;22: 181-7.

21. Bogduk N. The innervation of the lumbar spine. Spine 1983;8:286-93.

22. Standring S. Macroscopic anatomy of the spinal cord and spinal nerves. In Standrin S (Ed). Gray's Anatomy: The anatomical basis of clinical practice. Churchill Livingstone, London, 2005;775-88.

23. Bowsher D. A comparative study of the azygous venous system in man, monkey, dog, cat, rat and rabbit. J Anat 1954;88:400-406.

24. Woollam DHM, Millen JW. The arterial supply of the spinal cord and its significance. J Neurochem 1955;18:97-102.

25. Willis RJ. Caudal epidural blockade. In Cousins MJ, Bridenbaugh PO (Eds.), Neural blockade in clinical anesthesia and management of pain. Lippincott-Raven Press, New York, 1998;323-42.

26. Manchikanti L. Role of neuraxial steroids in interventional pain management. Pain Physician 2002;5:182-99.

27. Raj PP, Shah RV, Kay AD, Denaro S, Hoover JM. Bleeding risk in interventional pain practice: Assessment, management, and review of the literature. Pain Physician 2004;6:3-52.

28. Horlocker TT, Wedel DJ, Benzon H, Brown DL, Enneking FK, Heit JA, Mulroy MF, Rosenquist RW, Rowlingson J, Tryba M, Yuan CS. Regional anesthesia in the anticoagulated patient: Defining the risks (the second ASRA Consensus Conference on Neuraxial Anesthesia and Anticoagulation). Reg Anesth Pain Med 2003;28:172-97.

29. Houten JK, Errico TJ. Paraplegia after lumbosacral nerve root block: Report of three cases. Spine J 2002;2:70-75.

30. Lewandowski EM. The efficacy of solutions used in caudal neuroplasty. Pain Digest 1997;7:323-30.

31. Aldrete JA, Zapata JC, Ghaly R. Arachnoiditis following epidural adhesiolysis with hypertonic saline report of two cases. Pain Digest 1996; 6:368-70.
32. Manchikanti L, Bakhit CE. Removal of a torn Racz® catheter from lumbar epidural space. Reg Anesth 1997;22:579-81.
33. Kim RC, Porter RW, Choi BH, Kim SW. Myelopathy after intrathecal administration of hypertonic saline. Neurosurgery 1988;22:942-5.
34. Lucas JS, Ducker TB, Perot PL. Adverse reactions to intrathecal saline injections for control of pain. J Neurosurg 1975;42:557-61.
35. Nelson DA. Intraspinal therapy using methylprednisolone acetate. Spine 1993;18:278-86.
36. Kushner FH, Olson JC. Retinal hemorrhage as a consequence of epidural steroid injection. Arch Ophthalmol 1995;113:309-13.
37. Bromage PR, Benumof JL. Paraplegia following intracord injection during attempted epidural anesthesia under general anesthesia. Reg Anesth Pain Med 1998;23:104-7.
38. Rathmell JP, Garahan MB, Alsofrom GF. Epidural abscess following epidural analgesia. Reg Anesth Pain Med 2000;25:79-82.
39. Manchikanti L, Pampati VS, Beyer CD, Damron KS, Cash KA, Moss TL. The effect of neuraxial steroids on weight and bone mass density. A prospective evaluation. Pain Physician 2000;3:357-66.

Twenty Nine

Epiduroscopy for Chronic Low-Back Pain and Radiculopathy

S Gupta, J Richardson

INTRODUCTION

Endoscopic surgical procedures are one of the most significant advances in modern medicine. The development of miniature endoscopic instruments has given us a better insight into the contents of the epidural space and has helped in targeted therapy in the spinal canal. It also allows us to diagnose and treat patients while awake and without the need for an open surgical incision. This results in reduced risk, less trauma, shorter recovery time and reduced cost.

Technical Requirements

Outpatient based endoscopy procedures require miniaturized instruments because the patient is awake and under light sedation during the procedure. For epiduroscopy we need high quality optics, a cold light source, flexibility, steerability and a system for constant administration of a distending medium of saline. All this has to be made with as small an outside diameter as possible and it is really in the last decade that these requirements have been met.

How does epiduroscopy differ from gadolinium enhanced MRI which is the best available method of imaging to identify fibrous tissue in the spinal canal?

Epiduroscopy is better than MRI scan in identifying nerve root vascularity, nerve root inflammation, nerve root sensitivity, identification of fibrous tissue, diagnostic localization of pain and therapeutic aspect of pain management.[1,2]

MRI scan is better than epiduroscopy in delineating nerve root anatomy, identifying disc prolapse, assessment of spinal canal size and exclusion of serious pathology.

Pathophysiology of Radicular Pain

For generation of radicular pain, ischemia and/or inflammation are necessary. The nucleus pulposus which contains Phospholipase A2 and other irritant chemicals can leak from damaged intervertebral discs and can initiate an inflammatory reaction in the nerve root/dorsal root ganglion and can also subsequently promote fibrosis. Studies have shown that application of nucleus pulposus material to the nerve roots slows down nerve conduction and impairs nerve function.[3-5] Cytokines present in the synovial fluid of the facet joints can leak due to rupture of the joint capsule and cause nerve root irritation. Trauma, ischemia, inflammation of the nerve root and surgery can promote fibrosis, which can alter blood and CSF flow and compromise nutrition of the nerve root.

Proposed Treatment Algorithm for Low-Back Pain with Radiculopathy

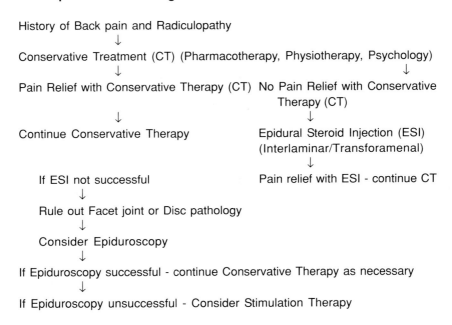

History of Back pain and Radiculopathy
↓
Conservative Treatment (CT) (Pharmacotherapy, Physiotherapy, Psychology)
↓   ↓
Pain Relief with Conservative Therapy (CT)   No Pain Relief with Conservative
                                                          Therapy (CT)
↓   ↓
Continue Conservative Therapy   Epidural Steroid Injection (ESI)
                                             (Interlaminar/Transforamenal)
                                                          ↓
If ESI not successful   Pain relief with ESI - continue CT
↓
Rule out Facet joint or Disc pathology
↓
Consider Epiduroscopy
↓
If Epiduroscopy successful - continue Conservative Therapy as necessary
↓
If Epiduroscopy unsuccessful - Consider Stimulation Therapy

Indications (Patient Selection)

Patients who have low-back pain with radiculopathy with no surgically correctable pathology on imaging and who have failed to respond to conservative management and epidural steroid injections are suitable for epiduroscopy. Before embarking on to epiduroscopy one should be convinced that the pain is not arising from the facet joints or the intervertebral discs.

Failed Back Surgery Syndrome (FBSS) is a term for patients who continue to have persistent back and/or leg pain even after surgery. It is a combination of severe nociceptive and neuropathic pains with superadded psychological component as treatment fails and time goes on. Between 5 and 50% of surgical interventions on the lumbar spine result in chronic pain. Approximately 37,500 patients with this syndrome are generated annually each year in the USA. As epiduroscopy can mobilize adhesions by mechanical and hydrostatic neuroplasty it may have a specific role to play for these patients without causing any further major trauma.

Contraindications

Contraindication for epiduroscopy include lack of consent, local infection at the sacral entry site, use of anticoagulants or a bleeding diathesis, hypersensitivity to amide local anesthetics or contrast media, pregnancy, marked obesity and uncontrolled hypertension. The patient needs to be able to lie prone for at least an hour.

How does SE Relieve Back pain?

The proposed mechanisms are that the saline flush helps in diluting and "washing out" of Phospholipase A2 and other irritant materials leaked from the intervertebral discs and the facet joints. Nerve roots with its inherent structural weakness, its poor blood supply and its nutritional reliance on CSF are easily engulfed by adhesions, compromising its nutrition. Epiduroscopy may improve nerve root nutrition and vascularity by breaking down adhesions. This is done by the saline flush used which helps in hydrostatic adhesiolysis (neuroplasty) and by mechanical adhesiolysis by the tip of the epiduroscope. Steriotactic placement of medications such as local anesthetic, steroid, clonidine and hyaluronidase provides targeted therapy. Studies have shown that upto 50% of epidural drug delivery may not be in the right place. Adhesions in the epidural space can prevent solutions reaching their target.

Epiduroscopy: Instrumentation and Procedure

Epiduroscopy is used for visualization and treatment of spinal canal. It is commonly performed via the caudal approach but the epidural space can also be visualized by carefully passing the spinal endoscope through a Tuohy needle at any level of the spine.

For epiduroscopy, patients are awake and in prone position with their feet inverted, as this improves access to the caudal epidural space. Soft pillows are placed under the patient as the procedure takes approximately one hour. The lumbar, sacral and caudal area is cleaned with betadine and draped as in any other surgical procedure.

In patients who are not allergic to penicillin cefuroxime 1.5 g is given I.V. as antibiotic prophylaxis.

Epidural Access Kit

Needles and syringes to inject local anesthetic into the skin, 18G Touhy needle, guide wire, dilator and epidural sheath (similar to pulmonary artery catheter sheath).

The procedure is carried out under midazolam sedation but a sensible verbal contact must be maintained with the patient during the entire procedure. Lignocaine 1% is injected into the skin over the sacrococcygeal area and the caudal epidural space is entered with an 18G Tuohy needle under lateral fluoroscopic guidance. Once the caudal epidural space is identified, radio-contrast dye is injected to obtain a baseline epidurogram. This may identify areas of filling defect that may correspond to the patient's symptom. A guide wire is then advanced into the epidural space through the Tuohy needle under fluoroscopy. The Tuohy needle is removed and a bold incision made at the entry point of the guide wire to facilitate smooth entry of the dilator along with the epidural sheath into the caudal epidural space. Adequate care is taken to prevent the guide wire becoming kinked. This is exactly as done when inserting a pulmonary artery catheter sheath in the intensive care unit (Figs 29.1 to 29.3).

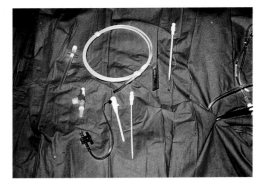

Fig. 29.1: Epidural access kit

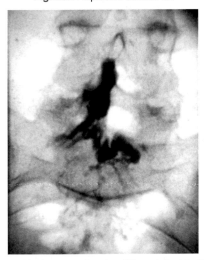

Fig. 29.2: Pre-procedure epidudrogram showing filling defect in the symptomatic right S1 nerve root area. There is also a filling defect around the right L4 and L5 area but this patient did not have any symptoms in the area supplied by right L4 and L5 and the filling defect was ignored.

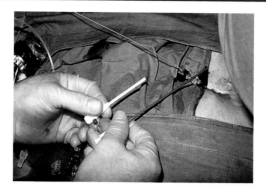

Fig. 29.3: Epidural needle with guide wire in place. The epidural sheath and the dilator are being assembled to pass over the guide wire into the caudal epidural space

Video Guided Catheter (VGC) or Steering Device

VGC is radiopaque and guides the flexible fiberoptic endoscope in the epidural space. The VGC we use is 2.7 mm in external diameter. It has two 1.3 mm working channels with a two-way steering mechanism and a radiopaque tip. The two working channels can be used; one for the fiberscope, the other for saline flush/instrumentation.

Side Port: There are two side ports that terminate with standard female luer locks. One side port is used for saline infusion and to monitor the epidural space pressure and the other port is left open to air to act as a vent for excess saline thus preventing excessive rise in epidural pressure.

Accessory Port: This port contains a Tuohy Borst adapter, duck bill valve, and side port channel. These ports are used to pass accessories through the working lumen of the catheter, i.e. fiberoptic scope, instruments.

Handle assembly: Houses the steering mechanism and is used to hold and direct the VGC.

Steering dial: Controls the steering mechanism that manipulates the tip of the VGC and thus the fiberscope can be directed in two different directions. This is exactly like using a fiberoptic bronchoscope.

VGC Shaft: Flexible shaft with steerable tip.

VGC distal tip: Radiopaque tip of VGC can be viewed under fluoroscopy (Fig. 29.4).

Flexible Fiberoptic Endoscope

The flexible fiberoptic endoscope works in conjunction with the VGC to provide direct visualization of the targeted pathology. The fiberoptic scope we use is 0.9 mm in external diameter and 125 cm long. Magnification is 40x and has a resolution of 10,000 pixels. It has a standard 32 mm eyepiece that couples to the video coupler. The distal tip incorporates the micro lens assembly.

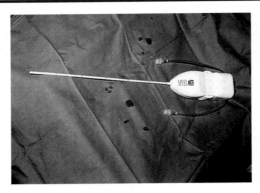

Fig. 29.4: The video guided catheter or the steering device with the handle which contains the steering device

The scope is connected to a cold light source and further connected to a video staking system to obtain images on the screen.

The flexible fiberoptic scope is passed through one of the lumena of the video guided catheter and threaded to project about 1 mm beyond the tip of the VGC. The side port of the VGC is connected to saline flush, which is hung about one meter above the level of the patient. A pressure-monitoring device may also be connected via a three-way tap to monitor epidural space pressure. It is important to keep the epidural pressure as low as possible and at least below the mean arterial pressure. Side effects such as headache, paresthesiae and back pain are directly proportional to the epidural space pressure.

The VGC along with the microendoscope is introduced into the epidural space through the epidural sheath. Saline is necessary for visibility and helps in hydrostatic adhesiolysis (neuroplasty). The tip of the VGC is guided towards the suspected sites of nerve root pathology under fluoroscopy. Hydrostatic pressure and movement of the tip of the VGC helps in releasing epidural adhesions and improves visibility and further spread of saline. With time, the epidural space clears and it will be possible to identify structures such as nerve roots. When the nerve root(s) responsible for the patients' symptom is touched, it produces exactly the same type and pattern of the patient's pain. After achieving satisfactory adhesiolysis and identifying the pathological nerve root, an epidurogram is performed and can be compared with the pre-procedure image. Generally a better spread of dye is noted. A steroid containing solution is injected at this site through one of the side ports of the VGC.

The VGC along with the fiberoptic endoscope and the epidural sheath is removed. The wound is covered with steri strips. The patient is kept supine for the next one hour and then discharged home (Figs 29.5 to 29.12).

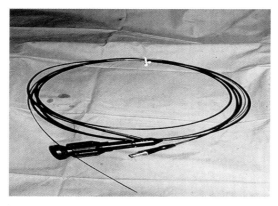

Fig. 29.5: The fiberoptic scope

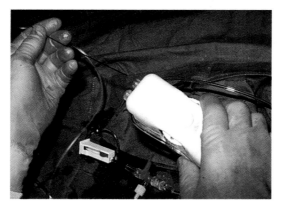

Fig. 29.6: The fiberoptic scope is being passed through the accessory port of the video guided catheter

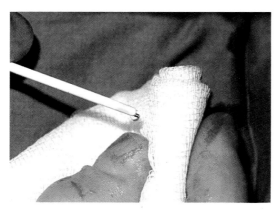

Fig. 29.7: The fiberoptic scope projects about 1 mm beyond the tip of the video guided catheter and is being focused

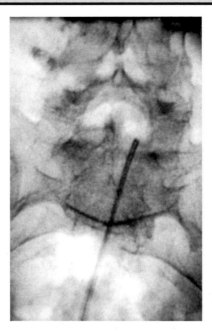

Fig. 29.8: The video guided catheter which houses the fiberoptic scope is guided to the suspected site of pathology under fluoroscopic and video guidance

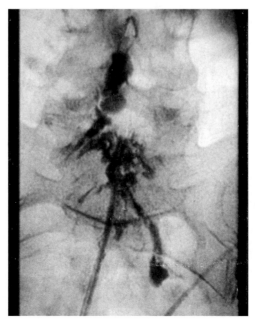

Fig. 29.9: Post procedure epidurogram showing good dye spread along the right S1 nerve root which was the pathological site in this patient

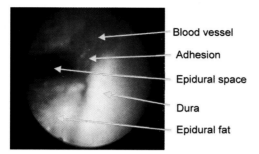

Fig. 29.10: Epiduroscopic picture showing adhesion which appear white, epidural fat which appear glistening, blood vessel, epidural space and dura

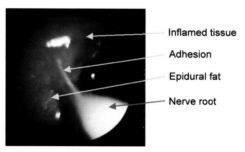

Fig. 29.11: Epiduroscopic picture showing inflamed tissue, adhesions epidural fat and nerve root

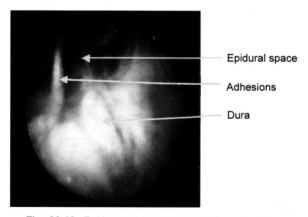

Fig. 29.12: Epiduroscopic picture showing adhesions

Sterilization Procedure for Fiberoptic Scope

NU-CIDEX: Contains 3500ppm peracetic acid. If the equipment is immersed in NU-CIDEX for five minutes it acts as a disinfectant and if immersed for ten minutes it sterilizes the equipment. Ethylene oxide gas sterilization can also be used.

Safety Considerations

Patient must be awake as they serve as their own monitor. Epidural space pressure due to saline infusion should not exceed mean arterial pressure.

The procedure should be stopped if patient reports pressure, paresthesia or complains of headache, ear-pressure, neck or shoulder pain as these symptoms indicate a rise in epidural space pressure. If these symptoms do not decrease the procedure may have to be abandoned.

Side Effects

Pain at the insertion site. Headache during or after the procedure. Small amounts of drainage from the epidural sheath insertion site. Paresthesiae during the procedure

Complications

Macular hemorrhage due to the transmission of epidural space pressure due to the hydraulics of CSF, dural puncture headache, epidural infection and/ or abscess, numbness, tingling, paresthesia, nerve root avulsion, meningitis, and arachnoiditis. To our knowledge there is no reported incidence of paralysis although this can be a potential complication.

Outcome Studies Following Spinal Endoscopy

As a general conclusion it may be said that about one third of patients derive significant pain relief and improved function after spinal endoscopy and another third derive no benefit from the procedure.[6-11] Geurts et al[7] concluded that 45% of their patients has >50% pain relief at[12] months following the procedure. There are several case reports suggesting favorable outcome following spinal endoscopy. However, Raffaeli et al[12] had 3 potentially lethal complications out of 10 patient examinations. These involved serious medullar irritation resulting in seizures, bradycardia and respiratory depression requiring emergency drug treatment and assisted ventilation. These events probably resulted from the large volume of epidural fluid that was used during the procedure (up to 1200 ml), as well as heavy sedation. Excess epidural space pressure is transmitted throughout the neuroaxis via the hydraulics of the CSF. The resulting intracranial pressures would have been very high. With our own examinations, lasting approximately one hour, we use approximately 100 ml of saline.

Conclusion

Back pain is a major problem in the society. No satisfactory treatment if yet available in all cases. The number of patients with Failed Back Surgery Syndrome is rising. If conservative measures or epidural steroid injections fail, epiduroscopy is a safe and effective day case treatment option in carefully selected patients who have low-back pain and radiculopathy.

Outcome results are encouraging although further studies are urgently needed. The use of laser[13] or radiofrequency co-ablation technique[14] to facilitate adhesiolysis in the epidural space appears promising.

REFERENCES

1. Igarashi T, et al. Thoracic and lumbar extradural structure examined by extraduroscope. Br J Anaesth 1998;81:121-5.
2. Igarashi T, et al. Inflammatory changes after extradural anaesthesia may effect the spread of local anaesthetic within the extradural space. Br J Anaesth 1996;77:347-51.
3. Otani K, Arai I, et al. Nucleus pulposus induced nerve root injury: Relationship between blood flow and motor nerve conduction velocity. Neurosurgery 1999;45 (3):614-9.
4. Olmarker K, et al. Pathogenesis of sciatic pain: Role of herniated nucleus pulopsus and deformation of spinal nerve root and dorsal root ganglion. Pain 1998;78:99-105.
5. Byrod G, Rydvik B, Nordborg C, Olmarker K. Early effects of nucleus pulposus application on spinal root morphology and function. European Journal of Spine 1998;7:445-9.
6. Richardson J, McGurgan P, Cheema S, Prasad R, Gupta S, et al. Spinal endoscopy in chronic low back pain with radiculopathy – A prospective case series. (MERIT Centre, Bradford Royal Infirmary. Anaesthesia 2001;56:454-60.
7. Geurts JW, Kallewaard JW, Richardson J, Groen GJ. (Rijnstate Hospital, Arnhem, The Netherlands and The MERIT Centre Bradford Royal Infirmary, Bradford, UK.) Targeted methylprednisolone acetate/hyaluronidase/clonidine injection after diagnostic epiduroscopy for chronic sciatica: A prospective, one-year follow-up study. Reg Anesth Pain Med 2002; 27(4): 343-52.
8. Igarashi T, Hirabayashi Y, Seo N, Saitoh K, Fukuda H, Suzuki H. Lysis of adhesions and epidural injection of steroid/local anaesthetic during epiduroscopy potentially alleviate low back and leg pain in elderly patients with lumbar spinal stenosis. Br J Anaesth 2004;93:181-7.
9. Manchikanti L, Pampati V, Bakhit CE, et al. Non-endoscopic and endoscopic adhesiolysis in post lumbar laminectomy syndrome. A one-year outcome study and cost effective analysis. Pain Physician 1999;2:52–8.
10. Manchikanti L, Rivera JJ, Pampati V, et al. Spinal endoscopic adhesiolysis in the management of chronic low back pain: a preliminary report of a randomized, double-blind trail. Pain Physician 2003;6:259–67.
11. Dashfield AK, Taylor MB, Cleaver JS, Farrow D. Comparison of caudal steroid epidural with targeted steroid placement during spinal endoscopy for chronic sciatica. A prospective, randomized, double-blind trial. Br J Anaesth 2005;94:514-9.
12. Raffaeli W, Pari G, Visani L, Balestri M. Periduroscopy. Preliminary reports – technical notes. The Pain Clinic 1999;11(3):209-12.
13. Ruetten S, Meyer O, Godolias G. Application of holmium YAG laser in epiduroscopy. Extended practicabilities in the treatment of chronic back pain syndrome. Journal of Clinical Laser Medicine and Surgery 2002;20(4) 203–6.
14. Raffaeli W, Righetti D. Surgical radiofrequency epiduroscopy technique (R-ResAblator) and FBBS treatment: Preliminary evaluations. Acta Neurochir 2005;92:121-5.

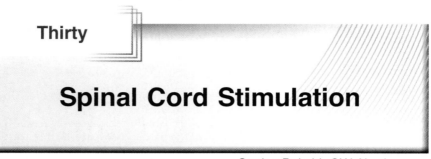

Thirty

Spinal Cord Stimulation

Sanjay Bakshi, GW Abrahamsen

INTRODUCTION

Chronic pain is often a difficult and costly condition to treat. In many cases, patients' symptomatology will fail to improve with traditional treatment modalities such as pharmacotherapy (NSAIDS, and neuropathic pain medications), physical therapy, chiropractic treatment, interventional spinal injections (epidural steroid injections, facet joint injections, sacroiliac joint blocks, stellate ganglion blocks, sympathetic blocks, etc.), and surgery. In these cases, treatment can be very frustrating for the clinician and patient and will often result in escalating doses of opioid pain medications.

At this point in a patient's treatment plan a clinician may consider modalities such as spinal cord stimulation (SCS). SCS has shown to be very effective and has been used worldwide for the treatment of angina, peripheral vascular disease, and chronic pain syndromes such as failed back syndrome, chronic, regional pain syndrome (CRPS), phantom limb, and arachnoiditis.[1-3] It is estimated that more than 250,000 neurostimulators have been surgically implanted since 1967.[4]

Spinal cord stimulation therapy blocks neuropathic pain by applying electrical stimulation over the spinal cord. This modality is most successful at alleviating neuropathic appendicular pain, but studies have also shown resolution of neuropathic axial pain.[5] SCS was first introduced in 1967 by Norman Shealy and colleagues.[6]

Mechanism of Action

The mechanism of action of spinal cord stimulation still remains controversial. The most commonly accepted mechanism is based on the gate control theory of pain published by Melzack and Wall in 1965.[7] This theory first proposed that painful "electrochemical" nociceptive information in the periphery is transmitted to the spinal cord in small-diameter, unmyelinated C-fibers and lightly myelinated A-Delta fibers. These fibers terminate at the substantia gelatinosa of the dorsal horn, the gate, of the spinal cord. Sensation such as touch and vibration is carried in large myelinated A-beta fibers and also terminate at this gate in the spinal cord. Therefore, the basis of this theory is that reception of large fiber information such as touch or vibration would turn off or close the gate to reception of small fiber information, resulting in analgesia.[8]

It has also been proposed that electrical stimulation may release putative neurotransmitters or neuromodulators, which effect prolonged pain relief.[9,10]

Indications

As mentioned earlier, SCS can be successfully used for many intractable pain conditions including angina, peripheral vascular disease, and chronic pain syndromes such as failed back syndrome, chronic regional pain syndrome (CRPS), phantom limb, and arachnoiditis. However, in the United States, the primary indications for SCS are failed back syndrome,[11] and complex region pain syndrome.[12-16] In contrast, in Europe SCS is commonly used as treatment for chronic intractable angina,[17-19] and peripheral vascular disease. SCS is also being used for pelvic pain, urologic disorders, occipital neuralgia and various other neuropathic pain conditions.

When considering SCS therapy the patient should have exhausted all conservative treatment modalities. The patient should also not be a candidate for corrective surgery which may alleviate the patients' symptoms. At this point a SCS trial may be considered using a multidisciplinary approach including neuropsychological screening to ensure appropriate patient selection.[20] Possible candidates for SCS therapy should also be reasonably intelligent to use the device, interpret their reduction of symptoms, and have good home support.

Contraindications

Neuropsychological clearance should rule out any underlying personality disorders, substance abuse, secondary gain issues, or unrealistic expectations from treatment that may alter the results from the trial. Other contraindications to SCS treatment include systemic infection, women who are pregnant or lactating, patients with a demand type cardiac pacemaker, coagulopathy, patients who experience discomfort from the sensation of TENS, and individuals who fail to achieve less than 50% reduction of pain during trial stimulation. After SCS has been implanted MRI and diathermy are also contraindicated.

Trial Stimulation

Prior to permanent implantation of SCS, all patients should undergo a trial. The most common trial method is a percutaneous trial, where leads are inserted into the epidural space percutaneously, and left in for a period of a few days to a week. At the end of the trial period, the leads are removed in the office by pulling them out of the skin. Some people prefer to do the trial by securing the leads in place surgically, and connecting it to a temporary extension that is externalized.

Some people also do an "on the table" trial. This trial only addresses the distribution of the stimulation pattern. It does not address the reduction of the patient's symptoms prior to permanent implantation of the device. For this reason, this method is infrequently used and may result in a higher rate of explantation of the stimulator device.

The patient should be assessed for a 50 to 70% reduction of the patients' typical pain, increase in the ability to perform activities of daily living, and possible reduction in patient's narcotic medication usage. Although spinal cord stimulation may reduce pain, it does not completely eliminate pain.[21-24]

The benefit of a SCS trial is that the patient can experience the sensation of stimulation and assess the percentage of pain relief prior to surgical implantation.

Surgical Implantation

Following a successful trial, planning for surgical implantation of the leads and generator should begin. As with any surgical procedure pre-operative clearance and informed consent should be obtained. Prior to the procedure the clinician should discuss with the patient a suitable implantation site for the pulse generator. It should be in a location that the patient would be able to reach with a remote to activate the device. Depending on operator and patient preference, the pulse generator or battery can be implanted in the flank, lower abdominal wall, or buttocks. Poorly placed pulse generators can lead to discomfort at the IPG site which may require surgical revision. The clinician will also need to decide whether to use a laminotomy or percutaneous lead. The other decision to be made is whether to have a standard or rechargeable battery.

Equipment

Currently, the three major manufacturers of spinal cord stimulation devices in the United States are Medtronics Inc., Advanced Neuromodulation Systems (ANS), and Advanced Bionics. The actual device should be decided on a case by case basis to suit individual patient's needs.

The basic components of the system are the lead, and the battery. The leads are percutaneous and laminotomy leads. The batteries are radiofrequency or externally powered, pulse generator or internally powered, and the new rechargeable batteries (Figs 30.1A to C).

Procedure

Step 1 – Trial Stimulation

Most often the trial is done percutaneously and this technique will be discussed here. The procedure described here is for placement of leads in the thoracic epidural space for treatment of back and leg pain. The patient lies on the table in the prone position with a pillow placed under the

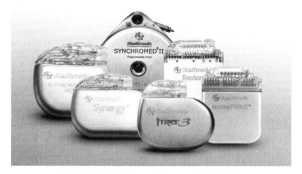

Fig. 30.1A: Different types of batteries
(Courtesy of Medtronic, USA)

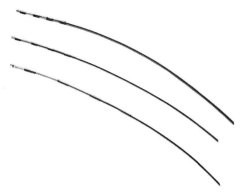

Fig. 30.1B: Different types of percutaneous leads
(Courtesy of Medtronic, USA)

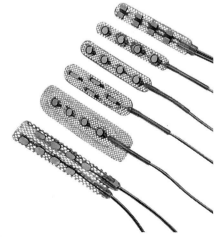

Fig. 30.1C: Different types of surgical leads
(Courtesy of Medtronic, USA)

abdomen. Mild sedation is used for the procedure. The procedure may be performed in a fluoroscopy suite or an operating room setting. Strict aseptic techniques are used. Antibiotics are given prophylactically before the procedure.

Initially fluoroscopy is used to count the levels. The author usually places a spinal needle across T10 so it serves as a landmark and you do not need to recount which level you are at. You can also make markings on the skin with a marking pen.

The entire procedure is done using fluoroscopy. Needle entry is usually at the T12-L1 level or L1-L2 level. Note that the angle of entry is much more shallow than a regular epidural. This makes it easier to thread the lead in the epidural space. It is preferable to first hit the lamina below to get an idea of depth. The needle is then walked off the lamina into the interlaminar space. Epidural space is identified using loss of resistance technique.

Once the epidural space is identified, the lead is inserted and threaded up to the T8 level. At this point you should check a lateral view to make sure the lead is in the posterior epidural space.

Sequential trialing is then done to check at which level patient gets appropriate coverage of the painful area. Depending on the patients pain distribution either 1 lead or 2 leads may be used. It is critical that the patient not be too sedated otherwise they will not be able to give you adequate feedback about their stimulation pattern if it is appropriately covering their area of pain.

Once you are satisfied that there is good overlap between the patients painful area and stimulation pattern, the needle is removed, with the lead left in place. After removal of the needle, make sure that the lead has not moved. This is done by comparing with the previous fluoroscopy picture. The lead is then fixed to the skin and sterile dressing is applied. Hard copies of the fluoroscopy films are saved for later reference during the permanent implantation.

At this stage the patient can be discharged home for an extended trial, or admitted for an inpatient trial depending on operator preference, and the patient's medical condition. If the patient is being discharged home it is advisable to observe the patient for a few hours after the procedure to make sure they do not develop any neurological deficits. Antibiotics are prescribed for the entire period that the leads remain in the patient during the trial. After the trial, the leads can be removed right in the doctors office. If the patient reports more than 50% relief of pain, and has improved activities of daily living during the trial period, they are considered appropriate candidates for a permanent implantation. Ideally they should use less pain medications during the trial period but that is not an absolute requirement for the trial to be considered successful (Figs 30.2A to F).

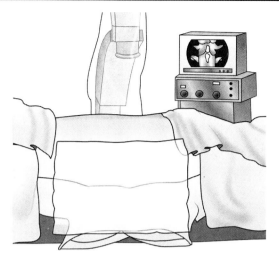

Fig. 30.2A: Initial position of patient
(Courtesy of Medtronic, USA)

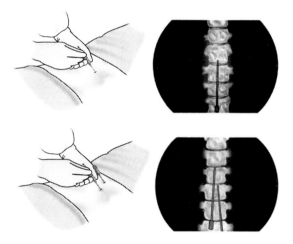

Fig. 30.2B: Needle entry percutaneous approach
(Courtesy of Medtronic, USA)

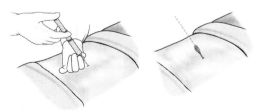

Fig. 30.2C: Loss of resistance technique
(Courtesy of Medtronic, USA)

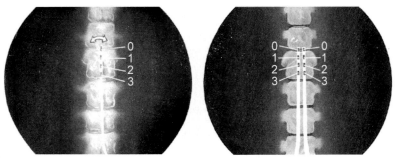

Fig. 30.2D: Fluoroscopic view of lead position
(Courtesy of Medtronic, USA)

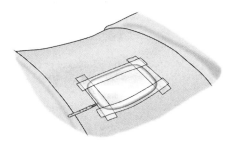

Fig. 30.2E: Sterile dressing applied at end of procedure
(Courtesy of Medtronic, USA)

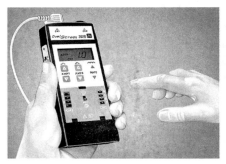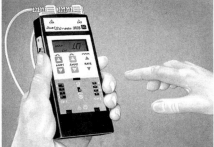

Fig. 30.2F: Programmer to check stimulation pattern
(Courtesy of Medtronic, USA)

Step 2 – Permanent Implantation

Once the patient is felt to be a successful candidate depending on the trial, the permanent implantation is performed. Prior to the procedure the implanting physician needs to have a detailed discussion with the patient about which type of battery would be appropriate, and the preferred site of implantation of the battery. The battery can be inserted in the flank, upper abdominal wall or the buttocks.

On the day of the procedure the battery site should be marked out in the holding area prior to the procedure.

On the operating table the patient is positioned in the prone position. Initial steps are exactly as for the trial.

Once the leads are in place, and the patient has appropriate coverage similar to or better than the trial, an incision is made around the lead, and dissected down to the supraspinous ligament. The lead is now anchored to the supraspinous ligament. This is probably the most important part of the procedure since the most common complication is movement of the leads. Therefore the leads need to be carefully secured to the supraspinous ligament.

The next step is the preparation of the pocket for the battery. The pocket is created so that there is adequate space for the battery as well as any excess lead or extension which needs to be tucked behind the battery. A radiofrequency generator should be generated no deeper than 1 cm below the skin, whereas a pulse generator is placed deeper, but no deeper than 1 inch below skin.

Once the pocket is created, tunneling is done between the pocket and the lead site, and the system is connected between the lead and the battery, either via an extension, or directly to the battery itself.

The entire system is checked at this point. If appropriate coverage is still present, the incisions are both closed in layers. Patient is usually discharged home the same day or the next day (Figs 30.3A to I).

Post-procedure Care following Surgical Implantation

Following surgical implantation, routine incision management and suture removal should be followed. Typically, the SCS is activated following removal of sutures. The patient should also refrain from any strenuous activity or reaching above the head until approximately 6 weeks. At this time the system is said to have matured, forming a fibrous capsule around the implant.

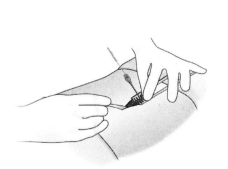

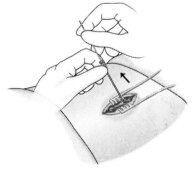

Fig. 30.3A: Incision around needle
(Courtesy of Medtronic, USA)

Fig. 30.3B: Needle removed – lead left in place
(Courtesy of Medtronic, USA)

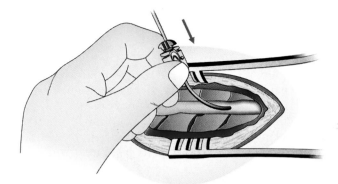

Fig. 30.3C: Anchor being threaded in
(Courtesy of Medtronic, USA)

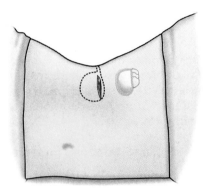

Fig. 30.3D: Pocket created for battery
(Courtesy of Medtronic, USA)

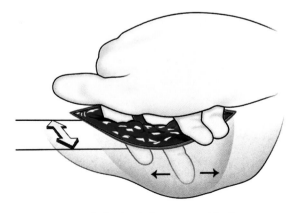

Fig. 30.3E: Pocket being prepared for battery
(Courtesy of Medtronic, USA)

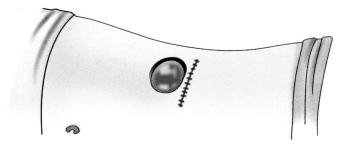

Fig. 30.3F: Tunneling between lead and battery site
(Courtesy of Medtronic, USA)

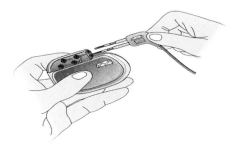

Fig. 30.3G: Battery being connected
(Courtesy of Medtronic, USA)

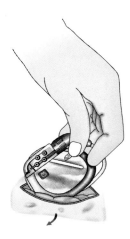

Fig. 30.3H: Battery being placed into
pocket *(Courtesy of Medtronic, USA)*

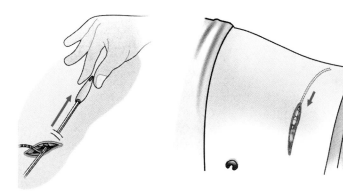

Fig. 30.3I: Incision closed in layers
(Courtesy of Medtronic, USA)

The patient should also have a thorough explanation on how to use the device. In some cases, the patient will have multiple programs and will require different degrees of stimulation throughout the day to achieve pain reduction.

Complications

Potential complications following SCS implantation include epidural hematoma, dural puncture headache, infection (including meningitis, epidural abcess), lead migration, pocket seroma, stitch abcess, and equipment failure.

The most serious complications are epidural hematoma and epidural abcess. Clinically, they are very rare, and can be minimized by meticulous surgical technique, and ensuring that the patients are not on any anticoagulation medication.

Dural puncture headache will typically resolve on its own, however, some patients may require an epidural blood patch for symptomatic relief. If a dural puncture headache occurs during a SCS trial it is recommended to abort the trial until resolution of the symptoms because the results of the trial may not be as accurate. Pocket seroma is an unlikely complication. This may require drainage if the seroma is severe or infected.

Lead migration is the most common complication following SCS implantation. When a lead migrates a patient will experience a change or complete loss of stimulation. Patients should be informed of the complication and the possibility of further surgical exploration to correct lead positioning.

Any part of the SCS system can fail at any point. Battery life is the most frequent issue. Numerous variables will affect the duration of battery life. These variables include the hours of use per day, the number of active electrodes, and program settings including amplitude, pulse width, and frequency. Newer pulse generators now have a rechargeable battery option, which may be considered in patients whose settings require more demand on the battery. However, patients should be informed that the rechargeable battery will also require replacement at some point.

Conclusion

Spinal cord stimulation can be a very valuable tool in the management of a wide variety of intractable chronic pain syndromes. It should be considered only when conservative measures have been exhausted and surgery is not a viable option. The success rate from this treatment modality can be high if performed with a multidisciplinary approach, in an appropriate candidate, using meticulous surgical technique, and with long-term follow-up.

REFERENCES

1. Vulink NC, Overgauuw DM, Jessurun GA, et al. The effects of spinal cord stimulation on the quality of life in patients with therapeutically chronic refractory angina pectoris. Neuromodulation 1999;2:33-40.
2. Claeys LG. Spinal cord stimulation and critical leg ischemia. Neuromodulation 1999;2:1-3.
3. Kumar K, Toth C, Nath RK, Laing P. Epidural spinal cord stimulation for treatment of chronic pain – some predictors of success. A 15-year experience. Surg Neurol 1998;50:110-21.
4. Industry estimates (Advanced neuromodulation systems and medtronic neurological), October 1999.
5. Law JD. Spinal stimulation: Statistical superiority of monophasic stimulation of narrowly separated, longitudinal bipoles having rostral cathodes.
6. Shealy CN, Mortimer JT, Reswick J. Electrical inhibition of pain by stimulation of the dorsal column. Preliminary clinical reports. Anesth Analg 1967;46: 489-91.
7. Melzack R, Wall P. Pain mechanisms: A new theory, Science 1965;150:971-8.
8. Krames ES. Neuroaugmentation. Mechanisms of action of spinal cord stimulation. Intervention Pain Management (2nd Ed) 2001; 53;561-5.
9. Levin BE, Hubschmann OR. Dorsal column stimulation: Effect of human cerebrospinal fluid and plasma catecholamines. Neurology 1980;30:65-71.
10. Meyerson BA, Brodin E, Linderoth B. Possible neurohumeral mechanisms in CNS stimulation for pain suppression. Appl Neurophysiol 1985; 48:175-80.
11. North RB, Ewend MG, Lawton MT, Piantadosi S. Spinal cord stimulation for chronic, intractable pain: Superiority of "multi-channel" devices. 1991; 44:119-30.
12. Oakley JC, Weiner RL. Spinal cord stimulation for complex regional pain syndrome: A prospective study of 19 patients at 2 centers. Neuromodulation 1999;2:47-51.
13. Bennett DS, Alo KM, Oakley J, Feler CA. Spinal cord stimulation for complex regional pain syndrome (RSD): A retrospective multicenter experience from 1995-1998 of 101 patients. Neuromodulation 1999;3:202-10.
14. Broseta J, et al. Chronic epidural dorsal column stimulation in the treatment of causalgic pain. Appl Neurophysiol 1982;45:190-94.
15. Barolat G, Schwartzman R, Woo R. Epidural spinal cord stimulation in the management of reflex sympathetic dystrophy. Stereotact Funct Neurosurg 1989;53:29-39.
16. Stanton-Hicks M. Spinal cord stimulation for the management of complex regional pain syndromes. Neuromodulation 1999;2:193-202.
17. Mannheimer C, Augustinsson LE, Carlsson CA, et al. Epidural spinal electrical stimulation in severe angina pectoris. Br Heart J 1998; 59:56-61.
18. Augustinsson LE. Spinal cord stimulation in severe angina pectoris: Surgical technique, intraoperative physiology, complications, and side effects. PACE 1989;12:693-4.
19. Murphy DF, Giles KE. Dorsal column stimulation for pain relief from intractable angina pectoris. 1987;3:365-8.

20. Olson KO, Bedder MD, Anderson VC, et al. Psychological variables associated with outcomes of spinal cord stimulation trails. Neuromodulation 1998;1:6-13.
21. North R, et al. Failed back syndrome: 5-year follow-up after spinal cord stimulator implantation. J Neurosurg 1991;28(5):692-9.
22. Kumar K, et al. Treatment of chronic pain by epidural spinal cord stimulation: A 10-year experience. J Neurosurg 1991;75:402-7.
23. Racz G, et al. Percutaneous dorsal column stimulator for chronic pain control. Spine 1989;14(1):1-4.
24. North R, et al. Spinal cord stimulation for chronic, intractable pain: Experience over two decades. J Neurosurg 1993; 32(3):384-95.

c. Specify lead : It has two, four electrode arrays spaced 2 mm apart, contact points are 2 × 3 mm and are spaced 6 mm apart vertically.

The pulse generator can be implantable (Itrel 3, Medtronic) or radio receiver based pulse generator with external stimulator (Xtrel, Medtronic). The battery life of implantable pulse generators depend on the use of the pacemaker, but usually last for an average of 4 to 5 years.

Surgical Technique

As with all implantable therapies, this consist of trial phase, followed by permanent implantation. There are two methods of placing the leads in epidural space. One is percutaneous method and the other is by open laminotomy. The percutaneous lead implantation is done under local anesthesia with sedation. Confirmation of the distribution and pattern of paresthesia is critical to a good outcome of SCS (Fig. 31.2). It has been observed that this is more important especially for patients requiring SCS for low back and radicular pain. However, if there has been a previous spinal surgery or the condition requires the use of plate electrodes (e.g. C1-C2 region) a laminotomy will need to be performed at the level of implantation and general anesthesia may be required.

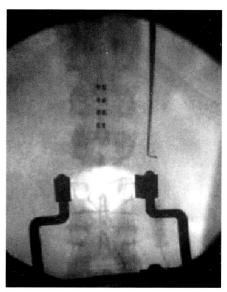

Fig. 31.2: Percutaneous lead electrodes for DCS in a patient with failed back surgery

Position of Electrode Insertion for Various Conditions

a. Occipital, jaw and neck pain: Electrode insertion at C1 and C2 level
b. Upper limb pain: Electrode insertion between C5 and T1
c. Lower limb pain: Electrode insertion between T9 and T11
d. For Angina pain: Electrode insertion between C7 and T1.

Following a successful screening period, the lead can be internalized and connected to the pacemaker. The implantable pulse generators come in mainly two different configurations. One is single channel (Itrel 3) and the other is dual channel (Synergy). It is possible to perform horizontal stimulation between two leads using synergy pacemaker. This is useful in axial pain syndromes and also to limit side effects.

Tolerance

Tolerance leading to decrease or ineffective stimulation remains a problem. It is caused by plasticity of pain pathways either in the spinal cord thalamus or cortex. Some times fibrosis around the stimulation tip can cause increase current thresholds. Minor lead displacements can be another reason for increased current requirements. Other factors like physiological, pathological and psychological factors may also be contributory to tolerance. One of the ways to overcome tolerance is by having stimulation "holiday" upto 6 weeks. In case of lead displacement or fibrosis, repositioning of the lead can be attempted.[24-26]

Complications/Adverse Effects of SCS
Descending Order of Frequency

1. Hardware failure: Displaced electrodes, fractured electrodes, IPG malfunction
2. Infection
3. Subcutaneous hematoma
4. CSF Leak
5. 90 degree rotation of pulse generator
6. Discomfort over pulse generator
7. Insulation damage
8. Spinal cord or nerve injury
9. Damage due to electromagnetic fields, e.g. diathermy, security system.

Results

The pain relief following SCS ranges from 50 to 60% in most reported series with failure or poor results in 30 to 36% patients. It has been documented that patients with failed back surgery syndrome respond better to spinal cord stimulation than the re-operation.[27] Reported success rates in treating failed back surgery syndrome vary from 12 to 88%, with higher efficacy reported in recent studies[28-30] systematic review of the literature related to spinal cord stimulation and failed back surgery syndrome by Turner et al [31] revealed that on average, 59% of patients had > 50% pain relief. The average complication rate in the same study was 42% but related to mainly minor complications. Besides pain relief, spinal cord stimulation improves functional status in a significant number of patients, with a 25% return-to-work rate[28] and up to 61% improvement in activities of daily living.[31] The reduced consumption of analgesics with spinal cord stimulation treatment varies from 40 to 84% in published reports.[32,33] Radicular pain responds more consistently than lumbar pain in patients with failed back syndrome. The initial response obtained in phantom limb pain patients can wear off over time. In patients with reflex sympathetic dystrophy the response rate in one of the large series.[34]

Conclusion

In the long run SCS is very cost effective compared to medical management. SCS provides significant long-term pain relief and improves the quality of life. Multipolar and Multichannel stimulation programs in SCS have improved the long-term success rate. In the present era complication rate is low which makes SCS relatively safe and effective approach for intractable pain management. Tolerance remains major problem in long-term course.

Motor Cortex Stimulation

The term "deafferentation pain" has been used to refer to pain in which the flow of afferent nervous impulses has been partially or completely interrupted.[35] Patients with deafferentation pain usually display sensory loss. The symptom common to all patients is a disturbance of temperature and pain sensibilities, whereas vibration and touch sensibilities may not be impaired.[36-38] There is increasing physiological evidence that nociceptive neuronal signal can be modulated by the input of non-noxious somatosensory information, such as light tactile sense, at multiple levels of central nervous system (CNS).[39,40] However, this modulation has to be done at a site above the level of deafferentation, e.g. deafferentation pain of peripheral nerve system can be effectively controlled by thalamic stimulation.[41-43]

Indications for MCS

1. Central neuropathic pain which has failed to respond adequately to medical therapy
2. Anesthesia dolorosa
3. Trigeminal deafferentiation pain
4. Central pain secondary to stroke. Severe motor deficit is a contraindication for MCS
5. Post herpetic neuralgia
6. Peripheral deafferentiation pain syndromes like brachial plexus or sciatic nerve injury
7. Spinal cord injury
8. Phantom limb and stump pain.

Mechanism of Pain Relief

Deafferentation pain secondary to CNS lesions, such as thalamic pain, has proved to be the most difficult pain syndrome to control even with stimulation therapy.[44-46] Pain control in such cases can be attempted by stimulating at a level more rostral to the thalamic relay nuclei. This is the basis for offering motor cortex stimulation (MCS). Tsubokawa and Katayama demonstrated that stimulation applied to precentral gyrus rather than the postcentral gyrus sometimes produced stronger pain inhibition. Stimulation of the postcentral gyrus even exacerbated pain in many patients. The area providing strong pain inhibition appeared to correspond to the motor cortex, since that area caused muscle contractions at higher intensity.[46,47]

Intact somatosensory cortex is not a prerequisite for the MCS but intact corticospinal tract neuronal system originating from the motor cortex is required for the pain relief to be effective. According to one study MCS attenuates brainstem spinal pain reflexes. Recent studies in such patient with functional MRI have shown that the cortical stimulation increases CBF in the ipsilateral thalamus, cingulate gyrus, orbitofrontal cortex and brainstem.

Surgical Technique

As with other stimulation therapies this also is a two staged procedure comprising of trial stimulation and permanent stimulation. Based on the MRI projections of the central sulcus a localized craniotomy is performed centered over it. The exact location of precentral sulcus is mapped using median nerve somatosensory evoked potentials. This is marked across the dura and the motor cortex is stimulate to elicit motor response (recorded by EMG and observing muscle contractions) in the areas of pain. Once the target site is confirmed the stimulating array of electrodes is replaced by a Medtronic Resume lead (Fig. 31.3). Trial stimulation is performed for 2 to 5

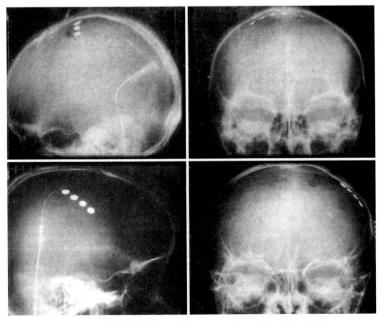

Fig. 31.3: Epidural electrodes for motor cortex stimulation

days. Stimulation parameters are frequency 40 Hz, pulse width 90 ms and amplitude 1 to 3 V. If there is more than 50% pain relief electrode is internalized and connected to an Itrel 3 pulse generator for permanent stimulation.

Results

The pain control rates in MCS ranges from 44 to 100%, depending on indications and technique.[48] The average pain control of more than 50% is achievable in >50% cases. Thalamic pain syndrome, post stroke pain, phantom limb pain and posttraumatic neuralgic pain (brachial plexus injury) have a better response. Patients may develop tolerance over long period of stimulation. This may be secondary to fibrosis in the epidural region around the electrodes or due to displacement of the electrodes.

Complications

1. Hemorrhage, infection as in any other surgery.
2. Risk of focal seizures due to motor cortex stimulation.

Conclusion

With the development in imaging technology and combination of functional MRI guided neuronavigation and intraoperative mapping has improved the targeting of motor cortex. Now studies have shown that patient's suffering with neuropathic facial pain of central and peripheral origins are greatly benefited. Emerging technology and innovation will bring better results in future.

REFERENCES

1. Thomas K Baumann. Physiologic Anatomy of pain. Youmans Neurological Surgery (5th Edn) 2917-36.
2. Kumar K; Hunter G, Demeria MD. Spinal cord stimulation in treatment of chronic benign pain. Challenges in treatment planning and present status, a 22 year experience, Neurosurgery 2006;58:481-96.
3. Fairbank JC, Davies JB, Couper J, O Brien JP. The Oswestry low back pain disability questionnaire. Physiotherapy 1980;66:271-3.
4. Melzack R. The McGill pain questionnaire: Major properties and scoring methods. Pain 1975;1:277-9.
5. Beck AT, Steer RA, Garbin MG. Psychometric properties of back depression inventory. Twenty five years of evaluation clin. Psychol Rev 1988;8:77-100.
6. Beck AT, Ward CH, Mendelson M, Mock J, Erbaugh J. An inventory for measuring depression. Arch Gen Psychiatry 1961;4:561-71.
7. Roland M. Morris R. A study of the natural history of back pain: Part I – Development of a reliabls and sensitive measure of disability in low back pain. Spine 1983;8:141-4.
8. Carlsson AM. Assessment of Chronic pain: Aspects of reliability and validity of visual analogue scale. Pain 1983;16:87-101.
9. Huskisson VC. Visual analogue scale, in Malzack R (Ed): Pain management and assessment. New York, Raven Press Inc. 1983;33-40.

10. Melzack R, Wall PD. Pain mechanism: A new theory. Science 1965;150:951-79.
11. Long DM. External electrical stimulation as a treatment of chronic pain. Minn Med 1974;57:195-8.
12. Meyer GA, Fields HL. Causalgia treated by selective large fibre stimulation of peripheral nerve. Brain 1972;95:163-8.
13. Turnbull Ian M, Shulman R, Woodhurst W Barrie. Thalamic stimulation for neuropathic pain. J Neurosurgery 1980;52:486-93.
14. Shealy C, Mortimer J, Reswick J. Electrical inhibition of pain by stimulation of the dorsal columns: Preliminary report. Anesth Analg 1967;46:489-91.
15. Dooley DM. Spinal cord Stimulation. AORN J 1976; 23(7): 1209-12.
16. Bell GK, Kidd D, North RB. Cost effectiveness analysis of spinal cord stimulation in treatment of failed back surgery syndrome. J Pain Symptom Manage 1997;13:286-95.
17. North RB, Nigrin DJ, Fowlewr KR, et al. Automated "Pain drawing" analysis by computer controlled patient – interactive neurological stimulation system. Pain 1992;50:51-7.
18. Alo KM, Yland MJ, Redko V, et al. Lumbar and sacral nerve root stimulation (NRS) in the treatment of chronic pain, a novel anatomic approach and neurostimulation technique. Neurostimulation 1999;2:19-27.
19. Linderoth B, Foreman R. Physiology of spinal cord stimulation: Review and update. Neuromodulation 1999;2:150-64.
20. Kumar K, Toth C, Nath KR, Verma AK, Burgess JJ: Improvement of limb circulation in peripheral vascular disease using epidural spinal cord stimulation. A prospective study. J Neurosurgery 1997;86:662-9.
21. DeJongste MJ. Spinal cord stimulation for Ischemic heart disease. Neurol Res 2000;22:293-8.
22. Erdek MA, Staats PS. Spinal cord stimulation for angina pectoris and vascular disease. Anesthesiol Clin North America 2003;21:797-804.
23. Foreman RD, Linderoth B, Ardell JL, et al. Modulation of intrinsic cardiac neurons by spinal cord stimulation: Implications for its therapeutic use in angina pectoris. Cardiovascular Research 2000;47:367-75.
24. North RB, Kidd DH, Zahurak M, et al. Spinal cord stimulation for chronic intractable pain: Two decade's experience. Neurosurg 1993;32:384-95.
25. Pineda A. Dorsal column stimulation and its prospects. Surg Neurol 1975;4:157-63.
26. Pineda A. Complications of dorsal column stimulation, J Neurosurge 1978;48:64-8.
27. Kolin MT, Winkelmuller W. Chronic pain after multiple lumbar discectomies – Significance of intermittent spinal cord stimulation. Pain 1990;5:S241.
28. North RB, Kidd DH, Lee MS, et al. Spinal cord stimulation versus reoperation for the failed back surgery syndrome: A prospective randomized study design. Stereotact Funct Neurosurg 1994;62:267-72.
29. North RB, Ewend MG, Lawton MT. Failed back surgery syndrome: Five year follow up after spinal cord stimulator implantation. A prospective, randomized study design. Neurosurg 1991;28:692-9.
30. Burchiel KJ, Anderson VC, Brown FD, et al. Prospective multicenter study of spinal cord stimulation for relief of chronic back and extremity pain. Spine1996;21:2786-94.
31. Turner JA, Loeser JD, Bell KG. Spinal cord stimulation for chronic low back pain: A systematic literature synthesis. Neurosurg 1995; 37:1088-96.

32. Burchiel KJ, Anderson VC, Brown FD, et al. Prospective multicenter study of spinal cord stimulation for relief of chronic back and extremity pain. Spine 1996;21:2786-94.
33. Kolin MT, Winkelmuller W. Chronic pain after multiple lumbar discectomies – Significance of intermittent spinal cord stimulation. Pain 1990;5:S241.
34. Giancarlo Barolat. Spinal cord stimulation for persistent pain management. In Textbook of stereotactic and functional neurosurgery, Gildenberg PL, Tasker RR (Eds), Mcgraw Hill 1998.
35. Tasker RR. Deafferntation, in Wall PD, Melzack R (Eds): Textbook of Pain. Edinburgh. Churchill Livingstone, 1984;119-32.
36. Holmgren H, Leijon G, Boivie J, et al. Central post-stroke pain–Somatosensory evoked potentials in relation to location of the lesion and sensory signs. Pain 1990;40:43-52.
37. Leijon G, Boivie J, Johansson I. Central Post-stroke pain–Neurological symptoms and pain characteristics. Pain 1989;36:13-25.
38. Pagni CA: Central pain due to spinal cord and brainstem damage in Wall PD, Melzack R (Eds): Textbook of pain. Edinburgh, Churchill Livingstone, 1984;481-95.
39. Fields HL, Adams JE. Pain after cortical injury relieved by electrical stimulation of the internal capsule. Brain 1974;97:169-78.
40. Hillman P, Wall PD. Inhibitory and excitatory factors influencing the receptive fields of lamina 5 spinal cord cells. Exp Brain Res 1969;9:284-306.
41. Gybles JM. Indications for the use of neurosurgical techniques in pain control, in Bond MR, Charlton JE, Woolf DJ (Eds): Proceedings of the VIth world Congress on Pain. Amsterdam, Elsevier 1991;475-82.
42. Hosobuchi Y. Subcortical electrical stimulation for control of intactable pain in humans. Report of 122 cases (1970-1984). J Neurosurg 1986;64:543-53.
43. Hosobuchi Y, Adams JE, Rutkin B. Chronic thalamic stimulation for the control of facial anesthesia dolorosa. Arch Neurol 1973;29:158-61.
44. Tasker RR. Deafferntation, in Wall PD, Melzack R (Eds). Text book of Pain. Edinburgh, Churchill Livingstone, 1984;119-32.
45. Tsubokawas T, Katayama Y, Yamamoto T, et al. Chronic motor cortex stimulation for the treatment of central pain. Acta Neurochir Suppl 1991;52:137-9.
46. Tsubokawas T, Katayama Y, Yamamoto T, et al. Deafferentation pain and stimulation of thalamic sensory relay nucleus: Clinical and experimental study. Appl Neurophysiol 1985;48:166-71.
47. Takashi Tsubokawa, Yoichi Katayama, Yamamoto T, et al. Chronic motor cortex stimulation in patients with thalamic pain. J Neurosurg 1993;78:393-401.
48. Helen Smith, Carlolf Joint, Daid Schlugman, et al. Motor cortex stimulation for neuropathic pain. Neurosurg Focus 2001;11(3):2.

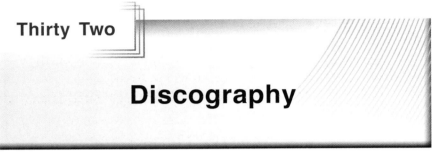

Thirty Two

Discography

Sudhir Diwan, P Annello

Introduction

Lindblom, in the 1940s, was first to describe a diagnostic disc puncture procedure, which he modified into what we call modern day discography. This procedure was previously used as an adjunct to myelography. Discography involves the injection of contrast into intervertebral discs to visualize any disruptions in the disc structure. Discography was further expanded to evaluate the patient's response to the injection in an attempt to reproduce the patient's pain. Modern discography has predominantely become a purely diagnostic modality, which can be utilized to obtain information in order to evaluate discogenic pain, and to determine the level of intervention or fusion.

Provocative discography is the term applied for the procedure to reproduce discogenic pain by injecting contrast in the disc. The pain is reproduced by two ways; first, by chemical irritation of sensitive tissue and secondly, by increasing the intradiscal pressure due to volume and stretching the annular fibers of the disc. Discography helps to evaluate disc morphology and confirm the diagnosis for consideration of surgical intervention. It also helps to confirm normal discs.

Why do Intervertebral Discs Cause Pain?

After extensive literature review it is believed that only the outer third of the annulus fibrosus has sensory nerve supply. But in case of internal disc disruption, there is ingrowth of sensory fibers into the inner third with neovascularization and neural expression of substance P. These ingrowths of nerve fibers play an important role in the pathogenesis of discogenic low back pain.[1]

At least one-third of patients with chronic low back pain have internal disc derangement (IDD). Disc degeneration is a progressive condition that gradually involves the entire nucleus and spreads radially to the annulus. IDD can happen with an intact annulus, and discography is gold standard to determine IDD.

Indications for Discography

- To confirm the source of pain in patients with a documented disc bulge.
- As a preoperative procedure to confirm the vertebral level for spinal fusion.
- Discography may help to distinguish source of pain either from the disc or scar tissue in postsurgical patients.
- In patients who are status post a fusion and continue to have persistent pain, discography can be used to see whether or not the discs adjacent to the fusion are the source of the patient's symptoms.
- To determine if other treatment modalities, e.g. IDET, nucleoplasty, chemonucleolysis would be of benefit for the patient's pain.[2,3]

Contraindications

- Patients unable to understand the procedure and unwilling to provide written consent.
- Systemic infection or localized infection at the site of procedure to be performed.
- Coagulopathic patient.
- Allergy to contrast medium.
- Significant myelopathic changes due to risk of aggravation of myelopathy.

Cervical Discography

Anatomy of Cervical Spine

- Cervical discs have certain characteristics distinct from other parts of the spine.
- Radicular pain originating exclusively from cervical disc herniation is much less common than in the lumbar region.
- The posterior longitudinal ligament in the cervical region is thicker, with a double layer, enclosing the posterior and lateral parts of the disc, while it is a much thinner, single layer, with weaker lateral protection in the lumbar area.
- The facet joints protect the cervical nerve roots from impingement by interposing a bony wall between the disc and the nerve root.
- The nuclear material of the cervical disc lies more anterior than it does in the lumbar spine, therefore posterior displacement is difficult to occur unless great forces are applied on the disc.
- The outer annulus is substantially thicker in the posterior portion of the cervical disc, making it more difficult for the disc to bulge posteriorly.
- Treatment of cervical discogenic pain is difficult because the disc receives sensory input from potentially different sources, and it is unclear which among them are responsible for pain.
- The anterior aspect of the disc receives sensory innervation from the sympathetic chain and the posterior aspect receives innervation from the sinovertebral nerves. It is thought that these nerves provide innervation to the facet joints as well.

Indications of Cervical Discography

There are several indications for performing cervical discography. These indications can be divided into those patients who have had a neurosurgical intervention or not.

- In surgical naïve patients, cervical discography is used to determine the source of pain in patients with documented evidence of a disc bulge on modern imaging studies like MRI or CT scan.[4]
- Discography may be used to reproduce pain in patients with persistent radicular pain but imaging studies may not show any anatomical abnormalities.
- Cervical discography can also be used as part of the preoperative workup for patients who are candidates for cervical fusion. It helps to determine the level of fusion by finding the disc that is most symptomatic and needs to be fused.
- Cervical discography can also be used to distinguish whether the etiology of a patient's pain is from a disc herniation or scar tissue.

Technique for Cervical Discography (Figs 32.1 to 32.5)

Fluoroscopic suite or operating room with C-arm fluoroscope is mandatory to perform the discogram at any level[5] (Fig. 32.3). The C-arm is rotated to 20 to 25 degree obliquely and angled cephalad or caudad to align the endplates of the intervertebral disc space.

- Prophylactic antibiotic should be considered.
- The patient is placed in the supine position with the neck in the neutral position.
- The right side of the neck is preferred due to the leftward orientation of the esophagus at this level. The neck is prepped and draped in the normal sterile fashion.
- Important structures must be noted at this level including the trachea, carotid artery, jugular vein and esophagus.
- The medial border of the sternocleidomastoid muscle is palpated and local anesthetic is injected subcutaneously at the chosen level of cervical disc.
- A 25-gauge, 3.5 inch styletted needle is placed through the skin and advanced to the middle of the disc in question.
- The needle is advanced incrementally with imaging. If a paresthesia is elicited, the needle should be withdrawn and then readvanced cephalad toward the middle of the disc.
- Once the disc is contacted, the needle is advanced incrementally under lateral view of the C-arm until the middle of the disc is penetrated.
- Imaging is performed in order to avoid going though the back of the disc either into the spinal canal or the pleura.
- 0.3 ml of contrast is injected with careful attention being paid to resistance to injection, patient's response and whether or not pressure is maintained or dissipated in the disc via manometery.[6]

- Make precise notes of amount of contrast injected, volume at which patient experienced pain, pressure at which patient experienced pressure/pain, and pain response (location, character, distribution, intensity and concordance with chronic pain).
- The discogram should be evaluated for the integrity of the disc and a decision should be made whether the adjacent disc needs to be studied or whether local anesthetic should be injected in the disc of question.
- The decision to inject local anesthetic into the disc space can give erroneous information if adjacent discs are to be evaluated. The local anesthetic can possibly track epidurally or it can anesthetize some of the nerves that provide sensory input to the adjacent discs.

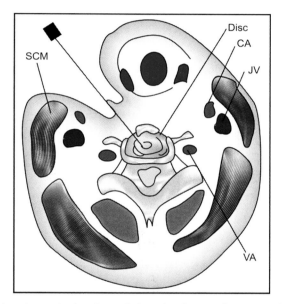

Fig. 32.1: Drawing demonstrating the technique for the anterior approach to the cervical disc. Abbreviations: SCM-sternocleidomastoid muscle, CA-carotid artery, JV-jugular vein, VA-vertebral artery

Imaging Details with X-ray

- The images of the injected disc should be evaluated to see whether or not the disc and its components are intact.
- The condition of the disc will determine where the contrast will collect.
- A normal disc will appear as a lobulated mass with some posterolateral clefts due to the normal aging process of the disc.
- If the inner annulus is torn, a transverse pattern of contrast will show on the nucleogram or if the tears of the annulus extend to the outer layer, a radial pattern will be noted.
- It is also possible for the contrast to flow into the epidural space or the endplate of the vertebra if the annulus is completely disrupted.

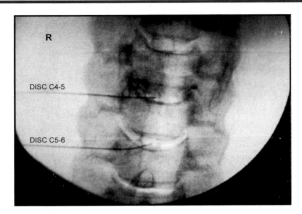

Fig. 32.2: X-ray imaging of cervical spine demonstrating entry of needles into C4-C5 and C5-C6 disc spaces

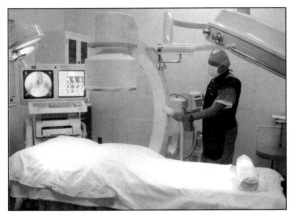

Fig. 32.3: Fluoroscopic suite with C-arm fluoroscope and fluoroscopic procedure table

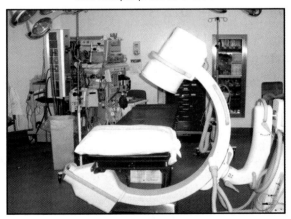

Fig. 32.4: Fluoroscope positioned for oblique view

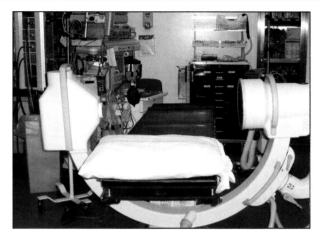

Fig. 32.5: Fluoroscope positioned for lateral view

- In certain situations, the injected contrast may flow between the layers of the annulus.

Anatomy of Thoracic Spine (Fig. 32.6)

- Thoracic discs are located between the cartilaginous endplates of the vertebrae above and below it.
- The disc of the thoracic spine is characterized by a thick fibroelastic annulus that surrounds a gelatinous nucleus pulposus.
- These annular fibers run in an oblique direction from adjacent vertebrae.
- These annular fibers receive sensory input from various sources including sinovertebral nerves (posteriorly) and the sympathetic chain (anteriorly).
- Nerve roots leave laterally through the intervertebral foramina.
- The disc can impinge the nerve roots if herniated laterally.
- The disc can impinge the spinal cord if herniated posterolaterally.

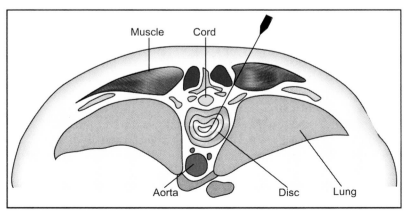

Fig. 32.6: Cross-section through thoracic area demonstrating entry point of styletted needle

Indications for Thoracic Discography

- Often most useful in determining source of pain but performed the least due to least likelihood of a thoracic disc to herniate.
- Patients with pain in whom testing have been normal or unrevealing.
- In postsurgical patients with persistent pain, one may want to differentiate scar tissue from disc tissue or evaluate the discs adjacent to a fusion.
- In presurgical candidates, discography may be used to further evaluate the levels to be fused.

Technique for Thoracic Discography

- Prophylactic antibiotics should be considered.
- Patient is placed in prone position with a pillow under the lower chest in order to flex the spine.
- If CT is being used, make careful note of pleura, lung, ribs, nerve roots and spinal cord.
- The spinous process above the disc of question is located and the skin 1.5 inches laterally on either side is prepped, draped and anesthetized.
- A 22-gauge, 3.5 inch styletted needle is placed through the skin and advanced to the middle of the disc of question.
- The needle is advanced incrementally with imaging. If a paresthesia is elicited, the needle should be withdrawn and then readvanced cephalad toward the middle of the disc.
- Once the disc is contacted, the needle is advanced incrementally until the middle of the disc is penetrated. Imaging is performed in order to avoid penetration of the back of the disc either into the spinal canal or the pleura.
- Similar to the cervical discogram, 0.3 ml of contrast suitable for intrathecal use is injected with careful attention being paid to resistance to injection, patient's response and whether or not a pressure is maintained or dissipated in the disc via manometry.
- Take note also of amount of contrast injected, volume at which patient experienced pain, pressure at which patient experienced pressure/pain, and pain response (location, character, distribution, intensity and concordance with chronic pain).
- The discogram needs to be evaluated to check the integrity of the disc and a decision needs to be made if there is need to evaluate the adjacent disc spaces or to inject local anesthetic in the disc of question.
- The decision to inject local anesthetic into this disk space can give erroneous information if the adjacent discs are to be evaluated. The local anesthetic can possibly track epidurally or it can anesthetize some of the nerves that provide sensory input to the adjacent discs.

Imaging Details with X-ray

- The images of the injected disc need to be evaluated to see whether or not the disc and its components are intact.
- The spread of the contrast will determine the condition of the disc.
- A normal disc will appear as a lobulated mass with some posterolateral clefts due to the normal aging process of the disc.
- If the inner annulus is torn, a transverse pattern of contrast will show on the nucleogram or if the tears of the annulus extend to the outer layer, a radial pattern will be noted.
- It is also possible for the contrast to flow into the epidural space or the endplate of the vertebra if the annulus is completely disrupted.
- In certain situations, the injected contrast may flow between the layers of the annulus.

Lumbar Discography (Figs 32.7 to 32.12)

Anatomy of Lumbar Spine

- Radicular pain of discogenic origin is much more common in the lumbar region than any other region.
- Unlike the cervical region, the bony facets do not protect the nerve roots.
- The posterior longitudinal ligament of the lumbar spine is thinner and less protective. This is especially true in the lateral aspects of the spine.
- The nuclear material in the lumbar spine is located more posterior than that of the cervical or thoracic spine.
- The nerve roots leave the spinal cord laterally and the laterally herniated disc can easily cause classic radicular symptoms.
- The innervation of the lumbar discs is very similar to that of the discs of the cervical and thoracic spine. The outer third of the annulus fibrosus of the disc is supplied by multiple sensory nerves.

Indications for Lumbar Discography[7]

- To determine source of pain in patients with documented disc bulge from previous studies.
- Patients with pain in whom testing have been normal or unrevealing.
- To differentiate scar tissue from disc tissue or evaluate the discs adjacent to a fusion in post-surgical patient with persistent pain.
- In presurgical candidates, discography may be used to further evaluate the levels needed to be fused.

Technique for Lumbar Discography

- Patient is placed in the prone position with a pillow under the abdomen to slightly flex the lumbar spine.
- Imaging can be obtained to locate vital organs like lungs, ribs, aorta, vena cava, kidneys, nerve roots, and spinal cord.

- The spinous process below the disc of question is palpated and the skin 1.5 inches laterally is sterilely prepped, draped and anesthetized with 1% lidocaine.
- A 22-gauge, 5 inch styletted needle is placed through the skin and advanced to the middle of the disc of question.
- The needle is advanced incrementally with imaging. If a paresthesia is elicited, the needle should be withdrawn and then redirected cephalad toward the middle of the disc.
- Once the disc is contacted, the needle is advanced incrementally until the middle of the disc is penetrated. Imaging is performed in order to avoid penetration though the back of the disc or too laterally either into the spinal canal or the pleura (in L1 discography).
- Similar to cervical discogram, contrast suitable for intrathecal use is injected with careful attention being paid to resistance to injection, patient's response and whether or not pressure is maintained or dissipated in the disc via manometery.
- Take note also of amount of contrast injected, volume at which patient experienced pain, pressure at which patient experienced pressure/pain, and pain response (location, character, distribution, intensity and concordance with chronic pain).
- The discogram needs to be evaluated to check the integrity of the disc and a decision needs to be made if there is need to evaluate the adjacent disc spaces or to inject local anesthetic in the disc of question.
- The decision to inject local anesthetic into this disk space can give erroneous information if the adjacent discs are to be evaluated. The local anesthetic can possibly track epidurally or it can anesthetize some of the nerves that provide sensory input to the adjacent discs.

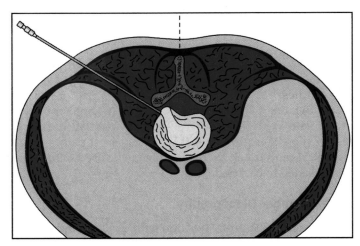

Fig. 32.7: Cross-section demonstrating the technique for lumbar discography. The needle is advanced toward the disc 8-10 cm from midline. The needle is angled 45 degrees from the surface of the skin

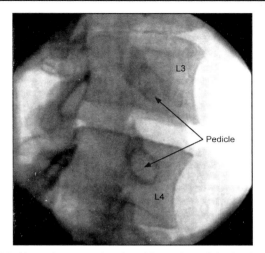

Fig. 32.8: X-ray demonstrating the oblique view of the lumbar spine. Refer to next figure for needle entry

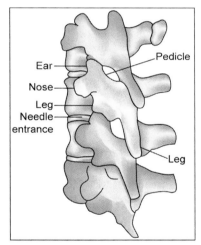

Fig. 32.9: Drawing depicting the "Scotty Dog" view of the lumbar spine. This figure can be used with the prior figure to determine exact point of needle entry

Imaging Details With X-ray

- The images of the injected disc need to be evaluated to see whether or not the disc and its components are intact.
- The condition of the disc will determine where the contrast will collect.
- A normal disc will appear as a lobulated mass with some posterolateral clefts due to the normal aging process of the disc.
- If the inner annulus is torn, a transverse pattern of contrast will show on the nucleogram or if the tears of the annulus extend to the outer layer, a radial pattern will be noted.

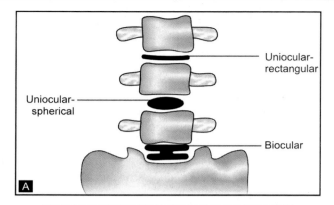

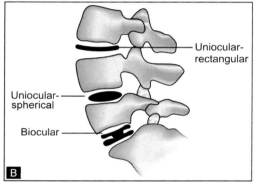

Figs 32.10A and B: Drawings depicting possible contrast flow after injection within the discs of the lumbar spine

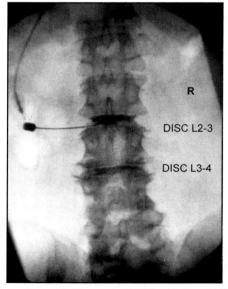

Fig. 32.11: X-ray demonstrating contrast in the L2-3 and L3-4 disc space

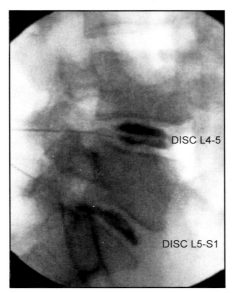

DISC L4-5

DISC L5-S1

Fig. 32.12: X-ray demonstrating contrast in the L4-5 and L5-S1 disc space

- It is also possible for the contrast to flow into the epidural space or the endplate of the vertebra if the annulus is completely disrupted.
- In certain situations, the injected contrast may flow between the layers of the annulus.

Side Effects and Complications of Discography

- Increased pain
- Headache
- Seizures
- Nausea
- Discitis (2-3% with single needle, 0.7% with double needle)
- Sympathetic block
- Diarrhea
- Urticaria
- Spinal headache
- Meningitis
- Intrathecal hemorrhage
- Arachnoiditis
- Epidural abscess/hematoma
- Trauma to nerve roots or spinal cord or cauda equina
- Allergic reaction to contrast
- Severe reaction to accidental intradural injection
- Damage to the disc
- Discography does not result in herniation of nucleus material or annular deterioration. Long-term follow-up studies have not demonstrated damage to normal disks after discography

- The incidence of discitis is 2-3% when a single-needle technique is used and 0.7% when a double-needle technique is used
- The incidence of discitis might decrease to less than 1% when prophylactic antibiotics are used
- The patient is instructed to ice the injection sites, and to call if they have any fever or any systemic signs of infection such as rigors, chills or shaking
- Pneumothorax (Upper lumbar, thoracic and lower cervical)
- Hemothorax (Upper lumbar, thoracic and lower cervical)
- Retroperitoneal hematoma (lumbar).

REFERENCES

1. Freemont AJ, Peacock TE, et al. Nerve ingrowth into diseased intervertebral disc in chronic back pain. Lancet 1997;350:178-81.
2. Derby R, Howard MW, et al. The ability of pressure controlled discography to predict surgical and non-surgical outcomes. Spine 1999;24-372.
3. Derby R and Lee SH. Discography? Intradiscal electrothermal annuloplasty. Pain medicine and management. Wallace MS and Staats PS (Eds.), Mc Graw Hill, New York 2005:350-53.
4. Sachs BL, Vanharanta H, et al. Dallas discogram description: A new classification of CT discography in low back pain disorders. 1987;12:287-94.
5. Schellhas KP, Garvey TA, et al. Cervical discography: Analysis of provoked responses at C2-3, C3-4 and C4-5. Am J Neuroradiol 2000;21:269-75.
6. Jarvik J, Deyo R. Diagnostic evaluation of low back pain with emphasis on imaging. Ann Intern Med 2002;137:586.
7. Guyer RD, Ohnmeiss DD. Contemporary concepts in spine care. Lumbar discography. Spine 1995;20:2048-59.

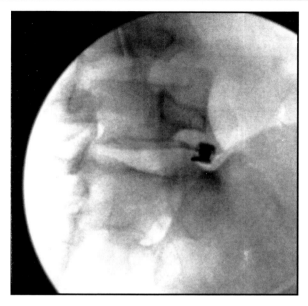

Fig. 33.2: This is an oblique fluoroscopy view. A needle is introduced and bony contact is made with the lateral aspect of the superior articular process to note the depth of insertion as well as to keep the needle as close to the superior articular process so as to avoid injuring the nerve root. Note that this procedure is being performed under end-on view

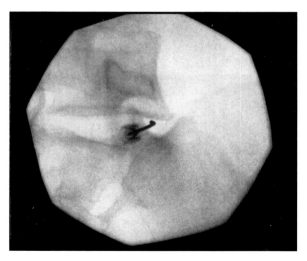

Fig. 33.3: The needle is slightly withdrawn and re-directed just lateral to the superior articular process. At this point, it is important to ask the patient if they notice any pain down the leg as the needle is advanced further. The resistance of the annulus is usually felt as the tip goes through the annulus and then the resistance goes away

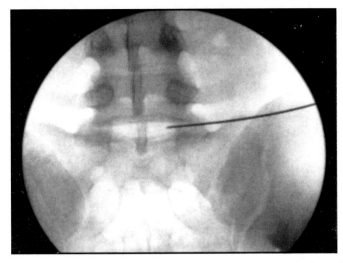

Fig. 33.4: AP fluoroscopy view. The needle tip is beyond the annulus into the nucleus, end-plates are lined up so as to make sure the needle is placed in the center of the disc space

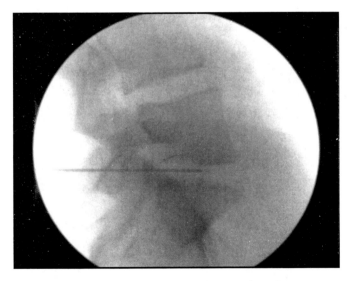

Fig. 33.5: Lateral fluoroscopy view, again noting the needle to be in the center of the disc space

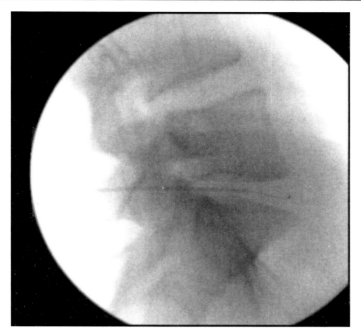

Fig. 33.6: IDET catheter is advanced under lateral fluoroscopy view. The two proximal and distal markers can be seen. The catheter is advanced and has started to curve back after contacting the inner annulus

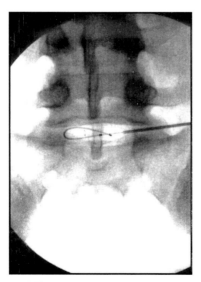

Fig. 33.7: AP fluoroscopy of IDET catheter is advanced further and can be seen wrapping around the posterior annulus. Both proximal and distal markers are out of the needle. At this point, the distal marker needs to be advanced slightly more so as to cover most of the posterior annulus

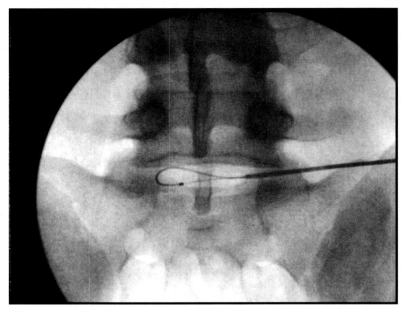

Fig. 33.8: The catheter is advanced further and both proximal and distal markers are lying along the posterior annulus from pedicle to pedicle. The distal marker is being shadowed by the introducer needle

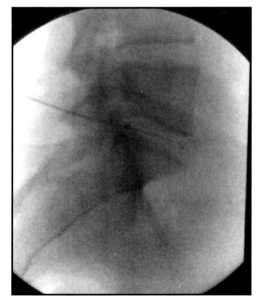

Fig. 33.9: Lateral view to confirm the catheter is not in the spinal canal

POST-OPERATIVE INSTRUCTIONS

The patient is to wear a brace for six weeks after the IDET procedure. An LSO lumbar brace is usually prescribed. The patient is instructed to limit their sitting from 30 to 40 minutes at a time for the first four weeks. They can perform sedentary activity one to three weeks after the procedure, but are to avoid excessive sitting. The patient can drive after the first few days, but the patient should limit driving time to 30 minutes. The patient is instructed not to lift more than 10 pounds for the first four weeks. They can walk 20 minutes daily and advance to 20 minutes twice daily after two weeks.

The patient is usually seen in our office two weeks after the procedure. Subsequent to that, their activity is increased slightly. At 6 to 8 weeks, they are sent for physical therapy, and resume daily activity with attention to back care and subsequent strengthening program.

COMPLICATIONS

Complications from this procedure can be related to the needle - injury of the nerve root, possibility of infection or discitis, and catheter tip breakage or dislodgement. Postoperatively, the patient can develop herniation if physical activity is not limited because of weakness of collagen fibers.[11]

There have also been cases reported of spinal cord injury and nerve root injury secondary to catheter misplacement, which was not diagnosed prior to the heating process.[9,10]

STUDIES RELATED TO IDET

In 1998, Saal and Saal presented 25 IDET patients. These patients underwent six months of conservative treatment followed by discography. The patients reported functional improvement and reduction of pain medicine. The initial study was not successful as it lacked control. Also, the researchers were the inventors of the IDET.

Saal and Saal published two-year follow-up data of 62 IDET patients.[12] Out of 62, 4 patients did not follow up in one year. The patients had the same inclusion and exclusion criteria. They were also excluded if they had any prior back surgery. At 24 months, the reported mean visual analog scale was 3.4 as compared to 6.5 pre-procedurally, 50% of the patients experienced a 4-point reduction in the visual analog scale and 71% patients experienced a 2-point reduction in the visual analog scale. They also showed improvement in quality of life. They did not report any complication in their study. This study was criticized for lack of randomization and lacks of control group as well as the investigators were the developers of this technology.

Bogduk and Karasek published a two-year follow-up study on IDET patients with chronic low-back pain.[13] Visual analog scale for pain, work status, and opioid use were used as outcome measures at three months. At three months, the pre-treatment median visual analog scale dropped from 8.0 to 3.4. At 24 months, 50% of IDET patient group had at least 50% relief of pain and 20% were completely pain free. The authors also concluded that the results are related to the catheter placement as close as possible to the annular tear and the fissures.

Lee et al. conducted a prospective non-randomized study in 62 patients with chronic low-back pain.[14] They also included patients who had prior discectomy. There was a statistical significant improvement in low-back pain. The study also was non-randomized and had no placebo control.

Pauza performed a randomized placebo control IDET study.[15] Uncompensated volunteers were selected. A total of 264 people were eligible. Patients were excluded from the study if they had any prior spine surgery, radicular pain, herniated disc, spinal stenosis, scoliosis, or narcotic usage greater than 100 mg of morphine. Also, the patients were excluded if they had workman compensation issues or personal injuries. A total of 64 patients were candidate for randomization. These patients underwent psychological testing, discography, and clinical examination.

The patients were randomized for IDET procedure or sham procedure. All the patients had the introducer needle introduced into the annulus. Randomized decision took place at the time of insertion of the introducer needle. The IDET group underwent standard heating of the IDET probe to 90 degree Centigrade. The sham group experienced the same visual and auditory environment as the treatment group. Following that, both groups were subjected to graded physical rehabilitation and follow-up was maintained for 12 months. Results showed 40% of patients treated with IDET experienced 50% or more pain relief, but 50% of patients experienced no notable improvement, 6% of patients showed worsening of pain, and 21% of patients showed greater than 80% reduction of pain.

SUMMARY

In general, IDET is a minimal invasive technique that shows significant promise for treatment of low-back pain coming from internal disc disruption or discogenic etiology, after receiving failed conservative treatments. It is a procedure which carries minimal risk if performed appropriately and suggests that half of the patients will notice significant improvement of back pain. The results are not as encouraging as they were with the initial studies, but this procedure is suggested to be performed on carefully selected patients who have primarily back pain and have undergone testing including discography and have not lost more than 80% of the disc height.

REFERENCES

1. Freemont A, Peacock T, Goupille P, et al. Nerve in-growth into diseased intervertebral disc in chronic low back pain. Lancer 1997;350:178-181.
2. Coppes M, Marani E, Thomeer R, Groen G. Innervation of painful discs. Spine 1997;22:2342-9.
3. Karasek M, Bogduk N. Intradiscal electrothermal annuloplasty: Percutaneous treatment of chronic discogenic low back pain. Tech Reg Anesth Pain Manage 2001;5:130-35.

4. Saal JA, Saal JS. Intradiscal electrothermal therapy for the treatment of chronic discogenic low back pain. Clin Sports Med 2002;21:167-87.

5. Sluijter ME. The use of radiofrequency lesions for pain relief in failed back patients. Int Disability Studies 1988;10:37-43.

6. Saal JA, Saal JS. Intradiscal electrothermal treatment for chronic discogenic low back pain: Prospective outcome study with a minimum 2-year follow-up. Spine 2000;27:966-74.

7. Heary R. Intradiscal electrothermal annuloplasty: The IDET procedure. J Spinal Disord 2001;14:353-60.

8. Narvani A, Tsiridis E, Wilson L. High intensity zone, intradiscal electrothermal therapy, and magnetic resonance imaging. J Spinal Disord Techniques 2003;16: 130-36.

9. Hsia A, Isaac K, Katz J. Cauda equina syndrome from intradiscal electrothermal therapy. Neurology 2002;55:320-28.

10. Djurasovic M, Glassman S, Dimar J, Johnson J. Vertebral osteonecrosis associated with the use of intradiscal electrothermal therapy: A case report. Spine 2002;27:325-8.

11. Cohen S, Larkin T, Polly D. A giant herniated disc following intradiscal electrothermal therapy. J Spinal Disord Techniques 2002;15:537-41.

12. Saal JA, Saal JS. Thermal characteristics of lumbar discs: Evaluation of a novel approach to targeted intradiscal thermal therapy. Presented at the 13th Annual Meeting of the North American Spine Society, San Francisco, CA 1998;23-8.

13. Bogduk N, Karasek M. Two year follow up of a controlled trial of intradiscal electrothermal anuloplasty for chronic low back pain resulting from internal disc disruption. Spine 2002;2:343-50.

14. Lee M, Cooper G, Lutz C, Hong H. Intradiscal electrothermal therapy (IDET) for treatment of chronic lumbar discogenic pain: A minimum 2-year clinical outcome study. Pain Physician 2003;6:443-8.

15. Pauza K, Howell S, Dreyfuss P, et al. A randomized placebo-controlled trial of intradiscal electrothermal therapy (IDET) for the treatment of discogenic low back pain. Spine 2004;4:27-35.

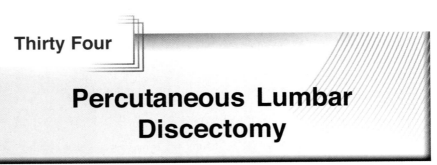

Thirty Four

Percutaneous Lumbar Discectomy

Sudhir Diwan, Dana Tarcatu

INTRODUCTION

It is estimated that 70 to 90% of all persons will experience low-back pain at some time in their lives. 80 to 90% will recover within about three months with physical therapy, medications, exercise and rest. However, some of these patients will go on to have chronic low-back pain.

Recently, a number of techniques have been developed that are applicable to the treatment of lumbar disc herniation and discogenic pain due to degenerative disc disease.

Pain generated by internal disc derangement is a relatively new concept. Several studies have demonstrated the presence of sensory nerve fibers in the annulus fibrosus of the disc and ingrowth of new nerves into degenerated discs in patients with chronic back pain.

These techniques have been designed either to shrink or remove disc material believed to be causing lumbar pain and/or radiculopathy. Studies have shown that by reducing the volume of disc, there is significant reduction in the intradiscal pressure that subsequently relieves the pressure over nerve roots. The most commonly examined and applied percutaneous techniques include arthroscopic microdiscectomy,[1] automated percutaneous lumbar discectomy,[2] percutaneous laser disc decompression[3-13] and chymopapain,[14,15] as well as other procedures.

General Criteria for Patient Selection

Persistent low-back pain for at least 6 months.
Patients have failed at least 3 months of aggressive non-operative therapy such as:
- Medications (NSAIDs, non-narcotic analgesics, narcotic analgesics, neural stabilizing medications)
- Injection therapy such as epidural steroid and facet injections
- Physical therapy.

Imaging in the Past Six Months Demonstrating

- At least 40 to 50% of the disc height preserved
- Annular tears
- No significant compressive lesion
- No significant central canal, neural foraminal, or lateral recess stenosis at the involved level
- Contained disc herniations.

Other Selection Criteria

- Concordant pain during provocative discography involving 1 or more discs
- Motivated patient with realistic expectations.

Contraindications

- Coagulopathy
- Severe radicular symptoms requiring surgery
- Previous disc surgery at the suspected level (relative contraindication)
- Imaging studies suggestive of nondiscogenic pathology
- Physiologic impairment that might interfere with post-procedure rehabilitation instructions
- Inflammatory arthritis
- Pregnancy
- Infection (systemic or local)
- Medical comorbidity that may affect appropriate follow up.

General Guidelines

Most procedures are performed in an operating room suite with the patient placed in a prone position on a standard operating table with bolster support (Fig. 34.1). This allows the use of fluoroscopy in which there is little radiographic obstruction. Local anesthesia is used in most of the cases. The C-arm fluoroscop is used to obtain anteroposterior, oblique ("needle eye view"), and lateral images (Fig. 34.2). Under strict sterile condition and fluoroscopic guidance, the appropriate disc level is localized. The so-called "Scotty dog" view is achieved by oblique fluoroscopic view.

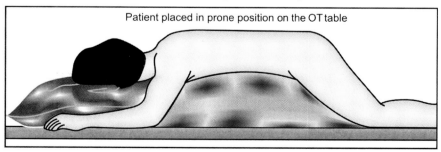

Patient placed in prone position on the OT table

Fig. 34.1: Diagram illustrating patient positioning for percutaneous discectomy

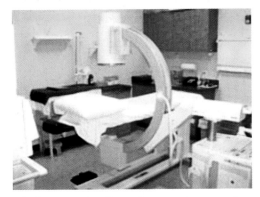

Fig. 34.2: Photograph demonstrating C-arm fluoroscopic use and operating room setup

Nucleoplasty

One of the commonly performed percutaneous procedure in the treatment of both discogenic low-back pain and radiculopathy secondary to contained disc herniation or disc bulge is nucleoplasty. It is a newer minimally invasive procedure that involves the percutaneous removal of disc material by using a co-ablation technique.

Specific Indications for Nucleoplasty Include

The indications for nucleoplasty include:
- MRI documented contained disc herniation or bulge
- Failed conservative treatment for more than 6 weeks
- Positive provocative discogram.

Contraindications

Complete disc space collapse leading to inaccessibility of the intervertebral space.
- Active disc space infection
- Medical conditions that would preclude its safe performance.
- Coagulopathy
- Spinal stenosis.

Equipments

- Perc-D wand (ArthroCare)
- ArthroCare power generator
- 17-gauge Crawford needle
- C-arm fluoroscope
- Fully equipped procedure room (operating room).

Procedure

Nucleoplasty involves the percutaneous insertion of a cannula positioned in the disc space. It is critical to have the best and safest approach to that area. Therefore, we usually use the anatomical triangular working zone described by Kambin, Parke, and O'Neill, et al. as landmark (Fig. 34.3). This "working triangle" avoids the exiting nerve root. The cannula is inserted on the same side as the patient's pain, i.e. the side ipsilateral to the disc herniation. The 17-gauge Crawford needle is used to access the disc and the Perc-D wand passes through the needle and appropriately placed in the center of the disc and midway between superior and inferior endplates. The wand is connected to ArthroCare power generator. Through the wand, the power and voltage are alternated to 125 V for ablation and 65 V for coagulation (Fig. 34.4 *upper* and *lower*). Approximately series of 6 channels are created within the disc to remove about 1 cc volume of nucleus pulposus. The procedure is performed under monitored anesthesia care in about 25 to 30 minutes.

The catheter has a low-temperature resister at its tip. The resister generates a plasma field that disintegrates disc material into its hydrogen and oxygen constituents. The gases escape through the needle (Fig. 34.5). A localized area of increased temperature may result in the ablation of adjacent residual disc material. The tissue ablation and thermal treatment create a series of channels within the disc, reducing the pressure from the contained disc herniation or the nerve root and other pain generating structures.

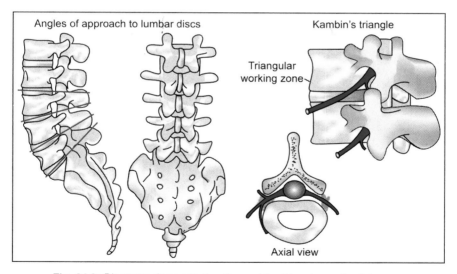

Fig. 34.3: Diagrams demonstrating the working triangles and safety zone for catheter placement

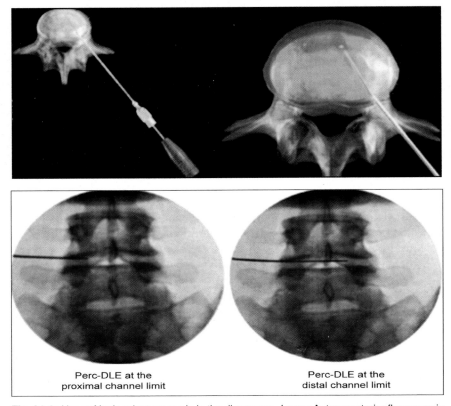

Perc-DLE at the
proximal channel limit

Perc-DLE at the
distal channel limit

Fig. 34.4: *Upper:* Nucleoplasty cannula in the disc space. *Lower:* Anteroposterior fluoroscopic image demonstrating placement of the nucleoplasty cannula in the disc space

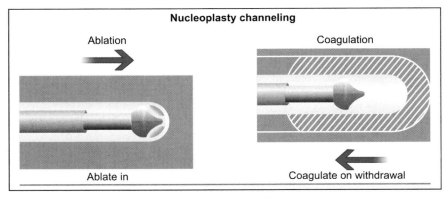

Fig. 34.5: Channeling during the nucleoplasty treatment

Dekompressor Discectomy

The Dekompressor probe (Fig. 34.6) manufacture by Stryker is disposable equipment intended for percutaneous discectomy. It is used to aspirate the disc material. Other than the probe, the placement of the introducer cannula, indications, contraindications are exactly the same as in nucleoplasty. The added advantage in this procedure is to visually appreciate aspirated disc material in the probe that can be sent for histological examination and for patient satisfaction.

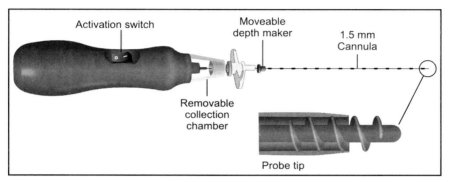

Fig. 34.6: Schematic presentation of dekompressor probe by stryker

Post-procedure Care

This is an ambulatory procedure that does not require any specialized care. Patient should rest for 2 to 3 days with limited ambulation, no strenuous work or bending. Lifting of 10 to 15 lbs only for 2 weeks. Physical therapy is indicated for at least 5 weeks. There is no need to wear a brace.

Outcome Results

Updated literature review supports that with increasing technical skills and improved equipment, nucleoplasty yields very positive results for relief of low-back pain and radiculopathy. Best results have been demonstrated in patients with diffuse disc protrusion and radicular pain, in whom good relief of radicular pain occurs almost immediately after the procedure.

Percutaneous Hydrodiscectomy

This is a newer technique in advancement of minimally invasive discectomy that involves fluid jet technology. The spinejet hydrodiscectomy system includes a microresector and access cannula set that uses power of water to cut the tissues and aspirate part of nucleus pulposus simultaneously. The fluid jet technology uses a high velocity stream of water to cleanly remove tissue. Anecdotal reports suggest that this technique may have a role in treating discogenic pain in selected group of patients. However, the benefits and risks of the procedure need to be evaluated by randomized trials to validate the effectiveness of the procedure.

Percutaneous Laser Disc Decompression (PLDD)

Choy and Diwan have done initial clinical research targeting YAG laser to reduce disc volume by vaporizing the disc. The laser was delivered in the center of the disc by an optical fiber through a 17-gauge introducer cannula. In vitro and in vivo studies have demonstrated sharp decrease in intradiscal pressure by decreasing the volume of the disc and subsequently taking pressure off of the compressed nerve root. However, this procedure did not achieve popularity due to expensive equipment and postoperative back spasms due to heat dispersion in the entire disc. Due to high potential for severe endplate and nerve root injury secondary to inability to control the heat dispersion, quest for least expensive, safer and minimal invasive technique continued.

Chemonucleolysis

Chemonucleolysis was the first technique used to percutaneously decompress the disc. In this approach, chymopapain, a proteolytic enzyme derived from latex of the papaya plant, is used to degrade a portion of the nucleus pulposus at the center of the disc. The use of chymopapain has virtually ceased in the United States due to several early instances of fatal anaphylactic reaction and acute transverse myelitis associated with its use. Though the chymopapain product is no longer marketed in the United States, chemonucleolysis continues to be popular, especially in Europe, due to its proven success rate and much improved management of allergic reaction when allergic pretesting is performed.

Nucleotome

Nucleotome was introduced in 1985. This automated shaver device mechanically withdraws nucleus pulposus from the disc in a procedure called "automated percutaneous lumbar discectomy" or APLD. The single use disposable APLD device is comprised of a reciprocating blade action, which draws disc tissue through a side-mounted port where it is subsequently aspirated from the disc. The device uses a 2.8 mm diameter cannula for disc access and does not require the use of an external controller. Again, this procedure did not become popular due to high cost and cumbersome nature of the equipment.

Summary

Internal disc disruption and contained disc herniations are common causes of low-back and/or lower extremity pain, which may become chronic if not diagnosed in a timely manner. Percutaneous disc decompression has been shown to be effective in relieving pain due to symptomatic contained disc herniation. Consideration of various complications and proper patient selection improve the chances of procedure success. Reherniation, instability, and potential for accelerated degeneration may be associated with percutaneous disc decompression procedures.

Despite the fact that percutaneuos lumbar discectomy has been around for almost 20 years, scientific proof of its efficacy still remains relatively poor. Well-designed research of sufficient scientific strength, comparing these techniques to both conventional surgery and conservative management of lumbar disk herniation is needed to determine whether percutaneous discectomy deserves a prominent place in the treatment arsenal for lumbar disk herniation.

REFERENCES

1. Yeung A. The evolution of percutaneous spinal endoscopy and discectomy: State of the art. The Mount Sinai Journal of Medicine 2000;67:327-32.
2. Onik G, et al. Automated percutaneous discectomy. Neurosurgery 1990;26: 228-32.
3. Choy DS, Diwan S. In vitro and in vivo fall of intradiscal pressure with laser disc decompression. J Clin Laser Med Surg 1992;10(6):435-7.
4. Singh V, Derby R. Percutaneous lumbar disc decompression. Pain Physician 2006;9:139-46.
5. Benz R, Garfin Steven. Current techniques of decompression of the lumbar spine. Clinical orthopaedics and related research 2001;384:75-81.
6. Singh K, Ledet E, et al. Intradiscal therapy: A review of current treatment modalities. Spine 2005; 30: s20-s26.
7. Sharps L, Isaac Z. Percutaneous disc decompression using nucleoplasty. Pain Physician 2002; 5:121-6.
8. Singh V, Pyrani C, at al. Percutaneous disc decompression using ablation (Nucleoplasty™) in the treatment of chronic discogenic pain. Pain Physician 2002; 5:250-59.
9. Pomerantz S, Hirsch J. Intradiscal therapies for discogenic pain. Semin Musculoskeletal Radiol 2006;10:2;125-36.
10. Fenton D, Czervionke L. Image-guided spine intervention 2003;10:257-83.
11. Welch W, Gerszten P Neurosurg Focus 2002;13(2).
12. McGraw K, Silber J. Intradiscal electrothermal therapy for the treatment of discogenic back pain. Applied Radiology 2001;30(7):11-6.
13. Choy DS, Diwan S, et al. Percutaneous laser disc decompression: A new therapeutic modality. Spine 1992; 17(8) 949-56.
14. Nordby EJ, Javid MJ. Continuing experience with chemonucleolysis. Mt Sinai J Med 2000; 67(4): 311-3.
15. Brown MD. Update on chemonucleolysis. Spine 1996; 21(24 Suppl): 62S-8S.

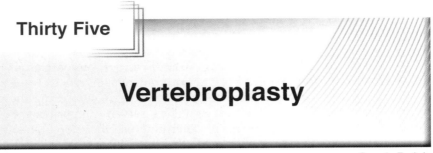

Thirty Five

Vertebroplasty

Samir Dalvie

INTRODUCTION

Percutaneous vertebroplasty was introduced in France in 1987 by Deramond[1] and Gailibert[2] for treating vertebral hemangioma. It is a simple, minimally invasive procedure for treating painful collapsed vertebrae. This procedure took some time to be established in mainstream medical practice, and was primarily used for tumor therapy in Europe for lesions such as multiple myeloma, lymphoma, metastatic disease and symptomatic benign tumors of the spine.[3] In North America, the first training course was held in 1998, and the primary use was for osteoporotic compressions fractures.[4,5]

Kyphoplasty[6,7] is a variation in the technique, where an inflatable balloon tamps is used to achieve partial fracture reduction and correction of kyphosis before cement injection.

Indications

In principle it is used for the treatment of painful vertebrae due to ostolysis. Indications in the clinical setting are as follows:

1. Osteoporotic vertebral compression fractures (VCF) (Fig. 35.1).
   More than 60% of post-menopausal women have abnormal bone mineral density, and 40% of these will sustain a vertebral fracture in their lifetime. There may be no history of definite trauma in 50%.

   Persistently painful fractures are associated with an increase in morbidity and mortality, with significant limitation of activities of daily living. Thoracic kyphosis is associated with a decrease in respiratory function.

   Non-operative management consists of bracing, analgesics and medical management of osteoporosis.

   Persistent pain may be associated with significant disability in activities of daily living, respiratory compromise and inactivity leading to venous thrombosis, etc. For many patients, a vertebral compression fracture represents the end of their independent life.

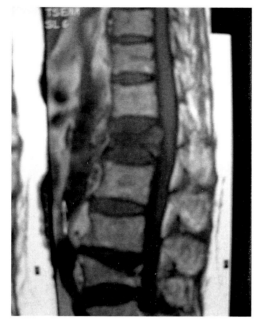
Fig. 35.1: MRI picture of compression fracture

Most vertebral fractures can be treated effectively by percutaneous vertebroplasty, with pain relief in 80 to 90% patients within 72 hours.

2. Malignant vertebral collapse

Pathological fractures due to malignant infiltration of vertebral bodies can be a cause of severe pain and disability. This includes metastasis from spindle cell tumors as well as hematological malignancies such as myeloma or lymphoma. Conventional treatment for palliation of pain consists of radiation along with analgesics, braces etc. More resistant cases may be subjected to major surgical procedures such as spinal stabilization or corpectomy and reconstruction.

Percutaneous vertebroplasty is an excellent, minimally invasive alternative with excellent results for pain relief. A filling of the lytic cavity caused by tumor infiltration is usually associated with excellent pain relief. Radiation therapy and vertebroplasty are complementary, and radiation should be performed after vertebroplasty.

3. Vertebral Hemangioma

Symptomatic vertebral hemangiomas can be treated with vertebroplasty, with or without prior instillation of ethanol. This amounts to cement embolization of the hemangioma, and produces good result. A transarterial angiogram and embolization is no longer considered necessary. In cases requiring surgical decompression due to progressive neurological symptoms, performing a vertebroplasty prior to surgical laminectomy is associated with reduced bleeding and complications.

Contraindications

1. Absence of proper indication.
2. Bleeding disorder.
3. Incompetence of posterior wall.
4. Vertebra plana. (complete collapse of the vertebra).
5. Sensitivity to local anesthetic, ingredients of bone cement.

Relative contraindications include improper set-up, inability to visualize radiologic anatomy adequately and severe medical disease with too many levels of involvement.

Mechanism of Action

The effects of vertebroplasty are primarily attributed to mechanical stabilization. The cement enters into the fracture planes, any cavities and into the interstices of the osteoporotic bones, and fuses these when the cement hardens. This would also abolish macro and micro motion on loading of the vertebrae.

Secondary mechanism could include ablation of the painful nerve endings by chemical and thermal effects of the setting cements.

Hemangiomas are addressed by filling of the venous channels with cement, thus permanently embolising them.

Procedure

The procedure is performed in an operating room or a fully equipped radiology suite. Essential equipment includes image intensification, if possible bi-plane, radiolucent adjustable table and equipment for monitoring vital parameters. A well trained and co-ordinated team consisting of technicians, nurses and an anesthetist makes the procedure simpler.

The procedure may be performed under local anesthesia with sedation or general anesthesia. Local anesthesia is preferred to restrict the morbidity of the procedure; however general anesthesia may be required in very apprehensive and un-cooperative patients or for multilevel procedures. I.V. access is mandatory, and I.V. antibiotics should be used prophylactically.

The patient is placed prone on the table on pillows or a radio-lucent mattress. The anatomy is defined with the C-arm. If the anatomic landmarks are not properly identifies, the procedure should be abandoned. The skin is prepared and draped in a sterile fashion.

Step 1 The entry point of the pedicle is marked on the skin by using crossed Kirshner wires, targeting the pedicle (35.2). For convergence of the needles, the skin entry-point should be slightly laterally placed. The skin is infiltrated with local anesthesia. Under lateral projection, the depth is infiltrated up to the periosteum.

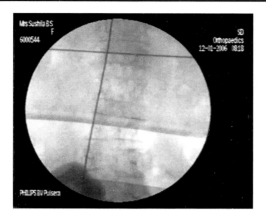

Fig. 35.2: Entry point on skin using Krishner wire

A stab knife is used to make a 4 mm incision in the skin. The procedure is performed with a bone biopsy (Jamshidi) needle, 11-gauges in the lumbar spine, and 13-gauge for the thoracic pedicles.

Step 2 Under fluoroscopic control, the needle is advanced into the pedicle, alternating the AP and lateral projections. Gentle hammering may be required if the bone is hard, else the needle is advanced by gentle rotation (Fig. 35.3). If the patient feels pain, I.V. sedation may be used at this point. I.V. midazolam and fentanyl are administered on an 'as needed' basis.

When the tip of the needle reaches the posterior cortex of the vertebra, the position is checked in the AP projection to make sure that the tip lies lateral to the medial wall of the pedicle.

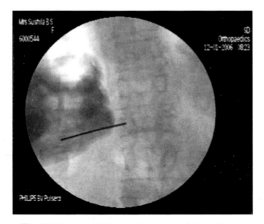

Fig. 35.3: Jamshidi needle into pedicle- AP view

Step 3 It is then advanced to lie in the anterior third of the body (Fig. 35.4).

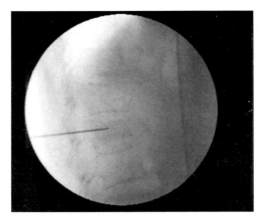

Fig. 35.4: Needle advanced deep into the body of vertebra

If bi-pedicular procedure is required, the same is repeated on the opposite side.

If required, and not contraindicated, non-ionic contrast may be injected at this point. This has however not been found to add value to the procedure and is now rarely performed.

Step 4 The cement is now prepared. Low or medium viscosity cement with added barium is used. The author uses Simplex or CMW3 bone cement. Barium powder which is previously sterilized is added to the powder. One teaspoon is added and mixed well. A teaspoon of the mixture is then removed to keep the amount of powder same. The liquid in then mixed well. When liquid, it is filled in a 20 cc syringe, which is then used to fill 1 cc syringes. The air is removed from these syringes. The consistency is then periodically checked. Ideal consistency must be similar to toothpaste, if it is too liquid there is a higher risk of leakage.

The stylet is removed, and cement injected slowly, with 0.2 cc increments under continuous fluoroscopic control (Fig. 35.5).

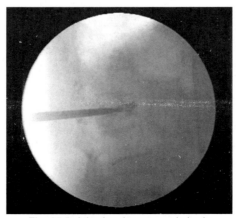

Fig. 35.5: Injecting the cement in body

It is mandatory to watch closely that the cement is not leaking into the surrounding tissue or vascular system. The stylet itself is used to gently push the cement as well as clean the needle. Alternate injections are made into each pedicle. The end point of injection is when the anterior third is filled, or if leakage starts.

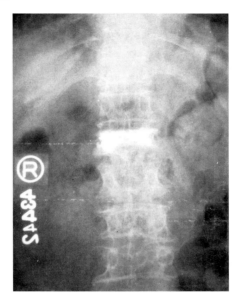

Fig. 35.6A: Cement in body of vertebrae- AP view

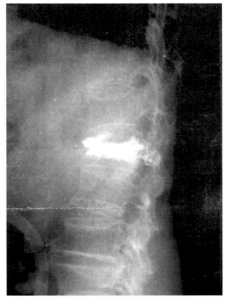

Fig. 35.6B: Cement in body of vertebrae- lateral view

Fluoroscopy must be confirmed in both planes (Figs 35.6A and B). Typically 2 to 6 cc of cement are required for each vertebra. Neurological monitoring can be carried out in the awake patients, and the patients should be asked about leg pain, which may be the result of intra-canal leakage.

The needles are left inside till the cement begins hardening, to prevent back flow of the cement through the needle tracks. After removal of the needle, the stab incisions may be secured with a suture, and dressed. The patient should be turned after the cement is fully hardened.

Post-operative Protocol

The patient may turn in bed, and can be made to sit 4 to 6 hours after the procedure. Analgesics may be required for the soft tissue pain. The patient can then be mobilized. Medical measures for control of osteoporosis are continued. The patient is encouraged to remain ambulatory and participate in activities of daily living.

COMPLICATIONS

Complication rates tend to vary with the underlying bone pathology as well as the experience of the operator. Published complication rates 1.3% in osteoporosis, 2.5% in hemangiomas and 10% in metastatic disease.

Cement embolism is the most dreaded complication, and can lead to morbidity and mortality. The cause is leakage of the liquid cement into the venous system para-vertebrally or epidurally.

Leakage of cement into the epidural space may cause neurological deficit related to spinal cord or root compression or radiculopathy. This may be due to a cortical breach in the posterior wall or filling of epidural veins. Such a complication may necessitate emergency decompressive surgery. Delayed cord compression may result from retropulsion of the cement mass, if there is collapse around the vertebroplasty.

Common complications include complications of positioning, notably a rib fracture. Uncommonly reported are deep infection, anaphylaxis and increased pain due to thermal necrosis

Long-term effects of the cement are as yet unknown; however there may be an increased incidence of adjacent level fractures related to increased stiffness of the cemented vertebra. Newer substances including hydroxy-apatite cement are under development to improve the biological acceptance of the construct.

RESULTS

Relief of back pain is the sole objective of percutaneous vertebroplasty. Various reports state the success rates as 80 to 90% for significant or complete reduction of pain from a vertebral fracture.

KYPHOPLASTY

Kyphoplasty is a variation in the technique of vertebroplasty. This involves introducing a balloon tamp into the vertebral body by a similar percutaneous route. This is inflated using normal saline under pressure. Expansion of the balloon causes the fractured endplates to be partially reduced, thus achieving a partial correction of kyphosis. It also creates a cavity, with a wall of compacted cancellous bone. The device is then deflated and removed. Bone cement is then injected into the cavity as with the vertebroplasty techniques.

Proponents of the kyphoplasty claim that its advantages include a fracture reduction as well as correction of the kyphosis. The creation of a cavity allows the cement to be injected at much lower pressures, and at a higher viscosity, and hence the chances of cement leakages are much lower. The disadvantages include a high cost of the disposable equipment, and longer treatment time, which may need a general anesthetic.

The available evidence does not suggest that the kyphoplasty has a clear advantage, as the pain relief is similar, and correction of kyphosis is not statistically significant. Cement leakage rates are lower than vertebroplasy, but the clinical complication rate is similar.

REFERENCES

1. Deramond H, Depriester C, Gailibert P. Percutaneous vertebroplasty with polymethylmethacrylate. Technique, indications and results. Radiol Clin North Am 1998; 533-46.
2. Gailibert P, Deramond H, Rosat P, Le Gars D. Preliminary note on the treatment of vertebral angioma by percutaneous acrylic vertebroplasty. Neurochirurgie 1987; 33: 166-8.
3. Barr JD, Barr MS, Lemley TJ, McCann RM. Percutaneous vertebroplasty for pain relief and spinal stabilization. Spine 2000;25: 923-8.
4. Voormolen MH, Mali WP, Lohle PN. Percutaneous vertebroplasty compared with optimal pain medication treatment: Short-term clinical outcome of patients with sub acute or chronic painful osteoporotic vertebral compression fractures. The VERTOS study. Am J Neuroradiol 2007;28(3):555-60.
5. Shen M, Kim Y. Osteoporotic vertebral fractures. A review of current surgical management techniques. Am J Orthop 2007;36(5):241-8.
6. Taylor RS, Taylor RJ, Fritzell P. Balloon kyphoplasty and vertebroplasty for vertebral compression fractures: A comparative systematic review of efficacy and safety. Spine 2006;31(23):2747-55.
7. De Negri P, Tirri T, Paternoster G, Modano P. Treatment of painful osteoporotic or traumatic vertebral compression fractures by percutaneous vertebral augmentation procedures: A nonrandomized comparison between vertebroplasty and kyphoplasty. Clin J Pain 2007; 23(5):425-30.

Thirty Six

Ozone and its Applications in Pain Management

Gautam Das

Since disc prolapse was first diagnosed by Dandy and subsequently by Mixter and Barr it has been implicated as one of the important cause of low-back pain radiating to limbs. Apart from conservative therapy all other forms of treatment aim at decompressing the nerve roots. These can be done by taking the disc out by surgery or by decompressing the foramen and disc by different interventions. The various treatment options have confused clinicians due to significant failure rate associated with different kinds of surgeries as well as with different interventions.

Outcome studies of lumbar disc surgeries document a success rate between 49 to 95% and re-operation after lumbar disc surgeries ranging from 4 to 15%. Reasons for this failure are: (1) dural fibrosis, (2) arachnoidal adhesions, (3) muscle and fascial fibrosis (4) mechanical instability resulting from the partial removal of bony and ligamentous structures required for surgical exposure and decompression (5) presence of neuropathy. There has been surge of interest in search of safer alternative method of decompressing the nerve roots maintaining the structural stability. Epidural steroid injection, transformational epidural procedures has a high success rate (up to 85%) but chances of recurrences are there specially if these interventions are done at later stage. Chemonucleolysis using chymopapain has also high success rate (approximately 80%) with low recurrences but not popular owing to the chances of anaphylaxis following intradiscal chymopapain injection. Injection of ozone for discogenic radiculopathy (low-back pain with radiation to legs) has developed as an alternative to chemonucleolysis and disc surgery owing to its high success rate, less invasiveness, fewer chances of recurrences and remarkably fewer side effects.

Muto[2-7] suggested intradiscal injection of ozone for disc hernia in 1998 under CT guidance. Leonardi popularized fluoroscopy guided ozone injection into the intervertebral disc. After that, successful outcome has been reported from various European centers. It is very important to note from those reports that complications are remarkably few. Not a single serious life-threatening complication was found even after 30,000 cases of ozone nucleolysis, which stresses the safety of these procedures.

How ozone acts? The action of ozone is due to the active oxygen atom liberated from breaking down of ozone molecule. When ozone is injected into the disc the active oxygen atom called the singlet oxygen or the free radical attaches with the proteo-glycan bridges in the jelly-like material or nucleus pulposus. They are broken down and they no longer capable of holding water. As a result disc shrinks and mummified and there is decompression of nerve roots. It is almost equivalent to surgical discectomy and so the procedure is called ozone discectomy or ozone ucleolysis. Besides, it has an anti-inflammatory action due to inhibitions of formation of inflammation producing substances; tissue oxygenation is increased due to increased 2, 3 diphosphoglycerate level in the red blood cells. All these leads to decompression of nerve roots, decreased inflammation of nerve roots, and increased oxygenation to the diseased tissue for repair work.

Indications

Ozone nucleolysis may be done in most kinds of disc related pain.
1. It can be done in degenerated disc without any prolapse and nerve root irritation. This category is called discogenic back pain. Dull ache in the low-back increasing with flexion of spine is the main clinical feature. Provocative discogram should be performed for this group.
2. It can be done in contained disc prolapse or disc bulge with root irritation.
3. It may be done in non-contained disc (extruded or sequestrated disc) as well.

Procedure

The patient is taken to the operation theater lying on prone position with a pillow under lower abdomen. The area is prepared and draped in sterile manner. It is done usually under local anesthesia with intravenous sedation (midazolam and fentanyl). Intravenous antibiotic like ceftriaxone 1G should be given prior to procedure. The procedure should be done under C-arm guidance. Though may be done under CT guidance.

Step 1 C-arm first should be focused to a pure anterior-posterior view to view the diseased disc. Then C-arm is cranially/caudally to abolish any double endplates and thereby getting widest possible view of disc space. Then C-arm is rotated obliquely away from vertebral column such that facet joint come at the center of the endplates (Fig. 36.1).

Now the needle entry point is just lateral to the superior pars/ articular pillar exactly at the center of the disc (Fig. 36.1).

Step 2 20 or 22 G needle is introduced into the diseased disc using tunnel vision (end on view, so that needle is seen almost as a single point) under fluoroscopic guidance (Fig. 36.2).

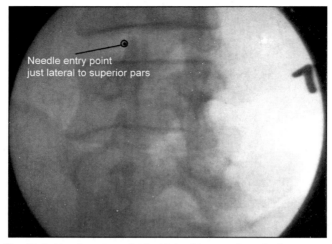

Fig. 36.1: Needle entry point just lateral to superior articular process

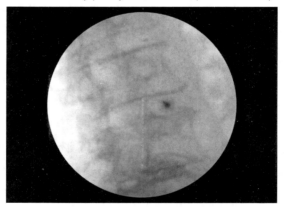

Fig. 36.2: Tunnel vision in lateral view

Step 3 The position of needle tip may be confirmed by complete AP and lateral view (Figs 36.3 and 36.4).

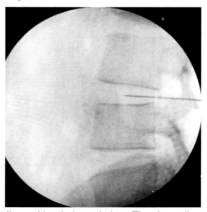

Fig. 36.3: Needle position in lateral view–Tip of needle at center of disc

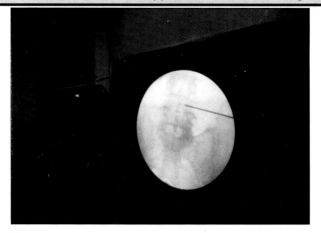

Fig. 36.4: Needle tip in AP view- Tip of needle in center of disc

Step 4 Some small amount of radiopaque dye (omnipaque) may be injected for discogram which is optional (Figs 36.5A, B and 36.6).

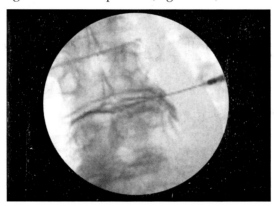

Fig. 36.5A: Discogram in AP view

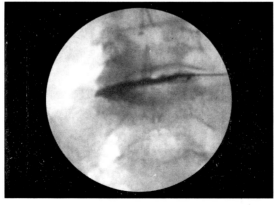

Fig. 36.5B: Discogram in AP view

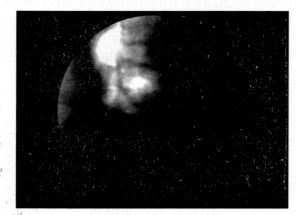

Fig. 36.6: Discogram in lateral view

Step 5 Then some 3 to 10 cc of oxygen-ozone mixture (at a concentration of 29-40 microgram/ml) is injected into the disc. Ozone at this concentration is not all harmful for the surrounded tissue. So if ozone spreads to the surrounded tissues including spinal cord, there is no harm. Ozone molecule is not stable. It has a half-life of 20 minutes only. So, within 20 minutes only half of the original ozone remains, the rest becomes oxygen. Increase in temperature decreases its half-life. For injection it is always freshly prepared on site (from an ozone generator) for immediate administration. Only ozone resistant syringes can be used for injecting it. While needle with the syringe is taken out some amount of oxygen-ozone mixture is also injected into the para-spinal muscle and para-radicular soft tissue to reduce nerve root inflammation and increased oxygenation of the para-spinal muscles.

Contraindications

There are few conditions when this procedure should not be performed. These are: active bleeding from any site, pregnancy, G6PD deficiency, active hyperthyroidism, loss of control of urination and defecation, and progressive sensory and motor loss.

Complications

Complications are very rare. They include post-procedural muscle spasm and burning pain (these are transient) and discitis (very rare due to the bactericidal effect of ozone). Other complications are similar to discographic procedure.

Ozone nucleolysis or ozone discectomy has a success rate of about 80%. On the other hand surgical discectomy has much higher side effects compared to remarkably few side effects of ozone discectomy. Ozone discectomy is usually a day care procedure and general anesthesia is not usually required. It is gaining popularity in different countries including India due to low cost, less hospital stay, fewer post-procedural discomforts and morbidity and very few side effects.

REFERENCES

1. D'Erme M, Scarchilli, Artale AM, et al. Ozone therapy in lumbar sciatic pain. Radiol Med 1998;95(1-2):21-4.
2. Muto M, Adreula C, Leonardi M. Treatment of herniated disc by oxygen-ozone injection. J Neuroradiol 2004;31:183-9.
3. Muto M, Avella. Percutaneous treatment of herniated lumbar disc by intradiscal oxygen-ozone injection. Interventional Neuroradiology 1998;4:273-86.
4. Vijay S Kumar. Total clinical and radiological resolution of acute, massive lumber disc prolapse by ozone nucleolysis. Rivista Italiana di Ossigeno-ozonoterapia 2005;4.
5. Nordby EJ, Fraser RD, David MJ. Chemonucleolysis. Spine 1996;21:1102-5.
6. Andreula CF, Simonetti L, De Santis, F et al. Minimally invasive oxygen ozone therapy for lumber disc herniation. Am J Neuroradio 2003;24:996-1000.
7. Torri G, Della GA, Casadei C. Clinical experience in the treatment of lumbar disc disease, with a cycle of lumbar muscle injection of an oxygen + ozone mixture. Int J Med Biol Env 1999;27:177-83.

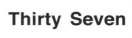

Thirty Seven

Radiofrequency Coagulation

Anil Sharma

HISTORY OF LESIONING OF NEVOUS SYSTEMS

Cryogenic Lesioning: Cryogenic lesioning has been used for cooling the tip of the probe to an extremely low temperature to freeze a region of tissue around the tip. This has been used for several years. The diameter of the probe is usually larger and duration of pain relief is shorter than other modalities.

Ultrasound: Ultrasound energy has also been used in the 1950s for lesions in the brain. It is difficult to control the size of the lesion, and also difficult to monitor the temperature.

Chemical Destruction: Injection of alcohol, phenol, or a glycerol has been used for peripheral nerve destruction. The disadvantage is not being able to control the flow of the injected material as a result the lesions are irregular, variable in size, and a significant chance of development of neuroma afterwards.

Lasers: Lasers have also been used to make lesions in the nervous system. It is difficult to quantify the extent and rapidity of tissue destruction using the laser and is not amendable to adequate temperature monitoring.

Radiofrequency Lesioning

Radiofrequency lesioning has been used since the 1950s, initially using continuous radiofrequency in the 1 megahertz range.[1,2]

Radiofrequency lesioning is generated by a radiofrequency generator, which is connected to the electrode placed in the body. The current flows between the tissues. The active electrode is positioned where the heat lesion has to be made and the other electrode is the large grounding pad, which is not intended to produce heat lesioning. The mechanism of the tissue heating is primarily ionic.[3] The radiofrequency voltage on the tip of the needle sets up electric fields in the space around the needle and the heat is generated. It is important to understand the tip of the needle does not actually heat up. The tip of the needle has a sensor, which gives a temperature reading. The equilibrium is usually reached in about 60 seconds. The size of the lesion depends on the electrode tip length as well as diameter and the temperature at the tip.

Radiofrequency denervation is a therapeutic procedure in which a Teflon-coated electrode with an exposed tip is inserted close to a nerve in such a manner that when a high frequency electric current is applied, it concentrates on the exposed tip and heats the immediate surrounding tissues and coagulates them.

LUMBAR RADIOFREQUENCY DENERVATION

This procedure is for the treatment of low-back pain originating from lumbar facet joint etiology. The rationale is based on performing diagnostic controlled blocks of medial branches that innervate the symptomatic joint, and the patient obtaining significant relief of back pain, up to 80%. Usually two sets of diagnostic injections are done. They can be done with a different duration of local anesthetic. After each diagnostic injection, the patient should report significant relief of back pain, which should be appropriate to the duration of local anesthetic used.

Anatomy of Medial Branches[4,5]

Medial branches of L1 to L4 dorsal rami all assume a similar course. Each medial branch crosses the base of the transverse process of the vertebra below, that is, a L3 medial branch crosses over the L4 transverse process and the L4 medial branches crosses over the L5 transverse process. Each nerve runs in a groove, which is formed by the junction of the transverse process and the superior articular process at each level. Each medial branch runs under the mamilla-accessory ligament[6] and it curves medially to enter the multifidus muscle. The ligament holds the nerve in place and there is little variation in the location of the nerve. Within the multifidus muscle, the medial branches divide into superior and inferior articular branches, which supply the relative facet joints above and below. As a result, each medial branch supplies two joints, that is, one joint is supplied by two medial branches. The segmental number of the joints innervated is not the same as segmental number of nerves that innervate them, so the L2 and L3 medial branch will innervate the L3-4 facet joint. The L5 dorsal ramus differs in its anatomy. It crosses over the most medial aspect of the ala of sacrum, and it is the dorsal ramus itself, which crosses the ala rather than its medial branch. It is located in the groove just lateral to the SAP of S1.

Principle of Radiofrequency Denervation

Radiofrequency denervation is performed by alternating a higher frequency electrical current between the larger surface area, which is the grounding pad, and a small surface area, which is the uninsulated tip of the needle. As the current approaches the electric tip, the electrical field becomes more dense and stronger and the current alternates causing the charged molecules to oscillate. Oscillation heats the tissue sufficiently to coagulate them. The volume of the coagulated tissue assumes the shape of a long spheroid whose long axis is formed by the uninsulated tip of the needle.

Coagulation occurs principally around the long axis of the needle that is sideways.[7,8] A very small amount of coagulation occurs distal to the tip of the needle. The size of the lesion and the dimension is proportional to the size of the electrode that is the length of electrode and the diameter of the electrode.

This concept about the lesion is important as placing the electrode perpendicular to the nerve will create a very small lesion and may quite miss it. Consequently, for optimal coagulation, electrode should be placed parallel to the nerve. Also, if smaller sized electrodes are used then multiple lesions have to be made.

The length of the sideway lesions is up to 1.6 to 2 electrodes distance. As a result of this, if multiple lesions are made, then the electrodes should be placed not more than one electrode distance between the consecutive placements.

Size of the lesion also depends on the duration of coagulation. As the temperature of the electrode reaches 65 degrees, coagulation starts on the surface. The volume of the coagulation tissue expands as the temperature increases to 80 degree Centigrade. At 30 seconds, the lesion increases to 85% of its maximum size. At 60 seconds, it reaches 94% of the size, which is attained at 90 seconds; thereafter increasing the time further does not increase the size of the lesion, so the optimal duration of coagulation is between 60 and 90 seconds.

The electrode of choice for lumbar radiofrequency is 150 mm, 20-gauge, long straight probe, with 10 mm active tip. Most common parameters are 80 degrees Centigrade for 90 seconds.

Patient Selection

The optimal patient for lumbar radiofrequency denervation is a patient with pain for at least three months with no indication of resolving by natural history. The pain has not responded to conservative treatment.

The pain is focal axial in nature, appears to be coming from facet joint etiology and has undergone controlled diagnostic blocks of the target medial branches with a different local anesthetic, done twice with each time the patient getting significant pain relief, greater than 80%.

Previous surgery does not preclude a successful response to percutaneous radiofrequency denervation and also can be done after recurrence of pain following previous radiofrequency denervation, as long as the duration of relief was more than one year.

The procedure is limited to minimal possible levels depending on the diagnostic test. The most common is three levels to denervate two facet joints. Coagulating more levels than that can cause greater portion of the lumbar musculature to be denervated.

Contraindications

Absolute contraindications to lumbar radiofrequency denervation are evidence of untreated infection, either systemic or at the proposed site, bleeding diathesis, patient is medically or psychologically unstable, as well as pregnancy.

Relative contraindications are patients with pacemaker and anatomical derangements that would compromise the safe placement of electrode, coexisting medical illness, immunosuppression, or unrealistic patient or family expectation.

Radiofrequency Denervation of Lumbar Medial Branches[9] (Figs 37.1 to 37.14)

Once the target points are identified under fluoroscopic guidance, the skin is anesthetized with local anesthetic and the probe is inserted. The electrode is placed parallel to the medial branches, so the C-Arm is tilted caudally and oblique to and the junction of SAP and transverse process is identified. It is always wise to make bony contact first, either at the inferior aspect of superior articular process or near the junction of the transverse process and the superior articular process. Once the depth is known, the needle is withdrawn slightly and readjusted to pass along the neck of the superior articular process by no more than a few millimeters. At this point, AP view of the placement is done which should show that the needle tip is against the lateral surface of the superior articular process. Subsequent to that, the lateral fluoroscopy view is obtained, which should show that the uninsulated tip lies along the middle of the neck of the superior articular process and the tip of the needle is appropriately away from the neural foramen.

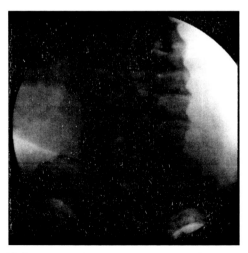

Fig. 37.1: This is an AP fluoroscopy view of the lumbar spine. The landmarks to be noted are the transverse process, the superior articular process, and the junction between those two. Also to be noted, this patient has spondylolysis at L5

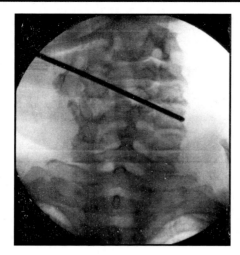

Fig. 37.2: Lumbar spine with caudal tilt of the C-arm, again noting the junction of superior articular process and transverse process. A needle is placed at an angulation so that they are parallel to the facet nerves

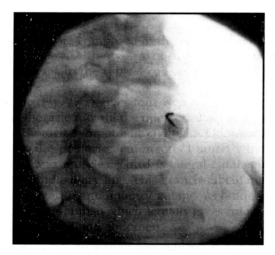

Fig. 37.3: After caudal angulation, an oblique view is performed, 15 to 20 degrees. Again, the landmark to be noted is the junction of superior articular process, transverse process, and the pedicle

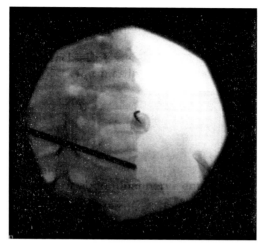

Fig. 37.4: Skin mark is placed at the junction of the superior articular process and transverse process, and a radiofrequency probe, 150 mm long with 10 mm active tip, is being introduced with the tip being directed towards the junction of superior articular process and transverse process

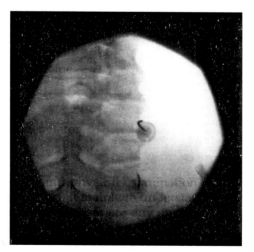

Fig. 37.5: This is in AP fluoroscopy view showing the radiofrequency probe lying in the gutter between the superior articular process and transverse process

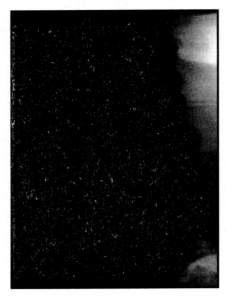

Fig. 37.6: The second radiofrequency probe of similar length is now placed at L4 facet nerve, again noting the junction of the superior articular process and transverse process. A bony contact is encountered and then subsequent to that, the needle slipped a few millimeters anteriorly

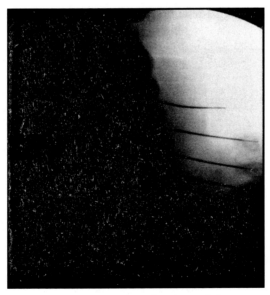

Fig. 37.7: This is in AP fluoroscopy view note that the radiofrequency probes are at the junction of the superior articular process and transverse process in the gutter. The active tip is lying parallel to the course of the medial branches

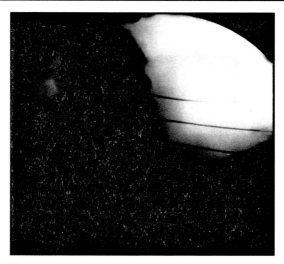

Fig. 37.8: Lateral fluoroscopy view showing the appropriate placement of the needles with the active tip lying along the lateral aspect of the superior articular process. Needle tip is posterior to the neural foramen

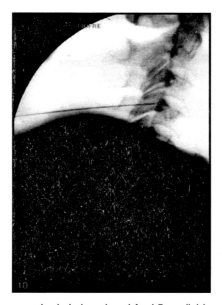

Fig. 37.9: Radiofrequency probe is being placed for L5 medial branch. This is performed under AP fluoroscopy guidance with slight cranial tilt to the C-arm. Usually the caudal tilt needed for lumbar facet nerves from L2 to L4 is not needed. The bony landmark is the superior articular process of S1, concavity or at the most medial aspect of the ala sacrum. A bony contact is made to determine the depth

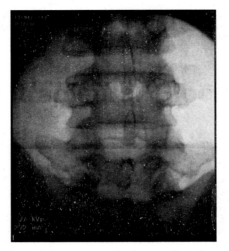

Fig. 37.10: The radiofrequency probe is now slipped anteriorly about 2 mm after bony contact is made

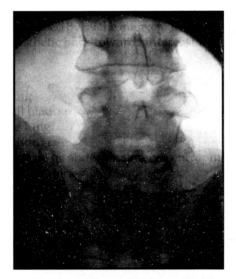

Fig. 37.11: Lateral fluoroscopy view is showing placement of radiofrequency probe for L5 medial branch

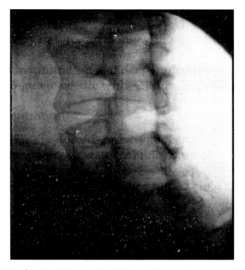

Fig. 37.12: Same patient with slight oblique view towards the left side to confirm the placement of the probes

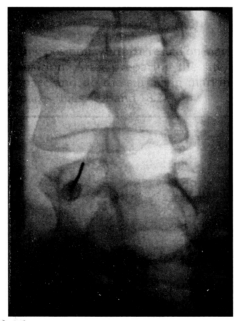

Fig. 37.13: This is in AP fluoroscopy view of patient undergoing L4 and L5 medial branch radiofrequency denervation

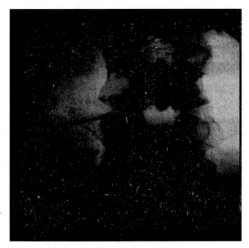

Fig. 37.14: Lateral view of the same patient

Once the fluoroscopy views are confirmed, then sensory testing for the medial branch is performed at 50 Hz. The current is slowly advanced in 0.1 increments and the patient is asked for reproduction of his back pain, pressure, or buzzing sensation in the back. Also, the patient is instructed to inform us if the pain starts to radiate in a radicular pattern down the legs. Usually with good placement, sensory stimulation is noted at less than 0.5 volts. Once the sensory testing is over, motor stimulation is carried out at 2 Hz, which should be done up to three times of sensory threshold. At this time, stimulation of paravertebral or multifidus muscles is usually noted, but there should be no motor stimulation of the lower extremities.

Once these parameters are noted and done at each level, 0.5 mL of 2% lidocaine is given through each needle to anesthetize the medial branch and radiofrequency coagulation is carried out. Usual setting is 80 degrees Centigrade for 90 seconds at each level.

Location of L5 dorsal ramus is different than the ones at L1 to L4 and the electrode is placed in not as much oblique or caudal direction. The target area is the most superior medial aspect of the ala area of sacrum, which is usually seen as a groove just lateral to the superior articular process of S1. Again, appropriate AP and lateral views should be obtained to check for the electrode placement relative to the neural foramen.

Once the procedure is done, 5 mg of kenalog mixed with 0.75% marcaine total 0.75 ml volume is injected at each level to decrease the incidence of post procedure pain and neuritis. The electrodes are removed. The area is cleaned and small bandages are applied. The patient is taken back to the recovery room. It is emphasized to the patient that they can experience numbness in the legs and that they must be careful when standing or walking immediately after the procedure because local anesthetic can track down to the segmental nerve root.

Post-operative Care

The patient is given detailed postoperative instructions including phone numbers in case of any problems. The patient is asked to apply cold packs for one to two days and to report any unusual symptoms including wound infection. Pain medications may be requested for a few days after the procedure. The patient is scheduled for a follow up visit two weeks after the procedure. Sometimes it could take up to three weeks for the patient to experience pain relief from this procedure. Initially they can develop neuritis or a hyperesthesia over the skin in the lower back where the medial branches provide some cutaneous supply. Rarely the symptoms can be quite bothersome, in those cases; trial of medications like gabapentin, topical lidocaine patch or cream can be beneficial for three to four weeks.

Complications of Lumbar Radiofrequency

Lumbar radiofrequency treatment is quite a safe procedure, but there are certain generic and theoretical risks, which are for any minimally invasive procedure. These include hematoma, infection, and allergic reactions. The placement of electrodes is done in such a way that it avoids any significant structure during insertion. Electrodes penetrate only the skin and posterior back muscles, and the spinal nerves lie anterior to where the electrodes are placed, so if the electrode is placed correctly there is no risk of nerve root injury. Also performing the procedure with less sedation will avoid any potential complications. The grounding plate has to be applied correctly otherwise there is a risk of skin burn. There is potential for increased pain as well as increased sensitivity of the skin, which a lot of patients complain as sunburn for up to 2 to 3 weeks after the procedure. If the symptoms are bothersome, then local lidocaine cream or patch can be applied and also occasionally gabapentin like medications can be prescribed to decrease the sensation.

RADIOFREQUENCY DENERVATION OF CERVICAL MEDIAL BRANCHES

Anatomy of Cervical Medial Branches[10]

The medial branches of the cervical dorsal rami course along the anterolateral and posterolateral aspect of the articular pillars. There is slight variation in the course of the medial branches depending on the level. At C5 level, the medial branch is along the middle fifth of the height of the articular pillar. The variation becomes greater at levels further away from the C5. For example, the C4 medial branch run relatively slightly higher along across the C4 articular pillar and the C6 medial branch will run slightly lower on the C6 articular pillar. The C7 medial branch is most often located crossing the superior articular process of C7. In an AP fluoroscopy view, the nerve is most often located on the corner formed by the junction at the C7 superior articular process and the root of the C7 transverse process.

At C3 level there are two medial branches, the C3 deep medial branch, which is involved in the nerve supply to the C3-4 facet joint and the C3 superficial medial branch, which is much larger and is also called the third occipital nerve and provides nerve supply to the C2-3 facet joints. In the lateral view, the C3 deep medial branch is usually running across the upper half of the C3 articular pillar. The third occipital nerve (the superficial C3 medial branch) crosses the C2-3 facet joint. In AP fluoroscopy view, the C3 deep medial branch is located slightly caudally into the upper half of the convexity of the C3-4 facet joint. The third occipital nerve is usually present into the lower half of the convexity of the C2-3 facet joints.

These variations in the location of the cervical medial branches need to be recognized for the proper application of radiofrequency denervation. The cervical medial branches are small targets and one needs to be more precise in the location of the needle to achieve an optimum result. The articular pillars are directed caudally and posteriorly so the electrode directed in that direction will place the exposed tip of the probe parallel to the medial branch.

If a direct anterior-posterior approach of the needle is used, then the lateral aspect of the superior articular process and any osteophyte coming from that will prevent the electrode from being placed directly on the nerve.

The third occipital nerve runs transversally across the anterolateral and lateral aspect of C2-3 facet joints. The electrode in that position can be placed without the caudal tilt.

Indication and Patient Selection

This is similar to radiofrequency denervation of lumbar facet nerves. The patient should have two diagnostic cervical medial branch blocks with different duration of local anesthetic with each providing around 80% relief of the pain.

Complications

Complications are similar to those of lumbar medial branch blocks. In addition, radiofrequency denervation of the third occipital nerve causes a numbness and neuritis in the occipital area and will also cause ataxia. Ataxia is not disabling. It amounts to the sense of potential unsteadiness. It is readily overcome if the patient uses vision to locate horizontal objects in the near or far distance.

Procedure for Radiofrequency Denervation of Cervical Medial Branches (Figs 37.15 to 37.23)

The patient is placed in the prone position with two pillows under the chest. My choice for cervical radiofrequency is from the posterior approach. While performing an AP fluoroscopy view, the mandible can obscure the good view of the concavities and articular pillars. The neck is rotated slightly to one side so as to remove the mandible shadow from the cervical spine. In

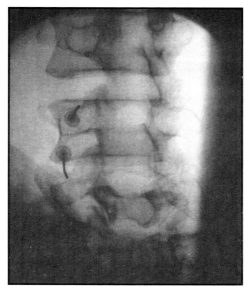

Fig. 37.15: This is an AP fluoroscopy view of the cervical spine. Please note the neck has been tilted slightly to the left side so as to avoid the mandible shadow from the cervical spine and because of this a very clear picture of concavities of the articular pillars are identified on the right side. The C-arm is also rotated caudally to obtain sharp view of concavities

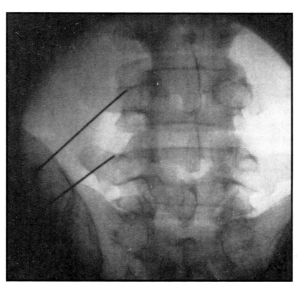

Fig. 37.16: A radiopaque marker is placed just lateral to the concavity of the C5 medial branch location

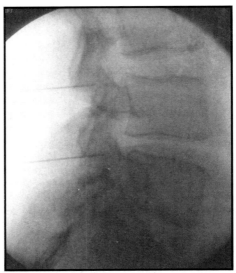

Fig. 37.17: A 100 mm long radiofrequency probe with a 5 mm active tip is introduced. A bony contact is made and then the needle is slightly withdrawn and slipped anteriorly for about 2 to 3 mm as can be seen on this fluoroscopy

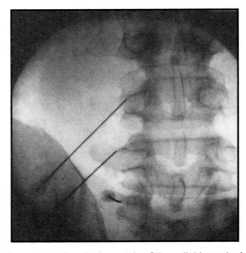

Fig. 37.18: This is a picture for placement for C7 medial branch. Again, a skin mark is placed at the junction of the transverse process and superior articular process of C7

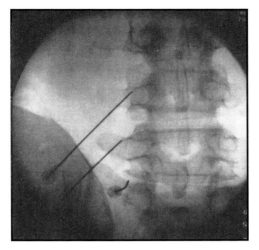

Fig. 37.19: A radiofrequency probe is placed along the previously marked site and bony contact is made

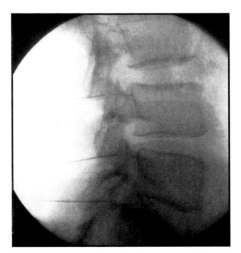

Fig. 37.20: Radiofrequency probes are placed with similar technique along C4, C5, C6, and C7 cervical medial branches. This is an AP fluoroscopy view

doing so, one must obtain a true AP fluoroscopy view by tilting the C-arm so that the spinous processes are placed into the center of the spine. After this the C-arm is tilted caudally to outline the articular pillars as identified by the concavities.

A skin mark is placed just lateral to the target concavity and the skin is infiltrated with 1% lidocaine. Following that, the radiofrequency probe is

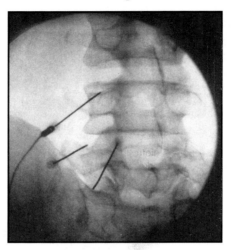

Fig. 37.21: Slight oblique view of the similar patient with the probes seen along the concavities

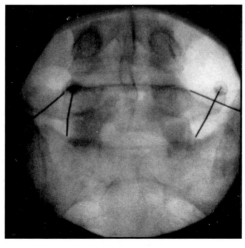

Fig. 37.22: Slightly more oblique view to look for the placement of the probe. It is noted that the tip of the needles are away from the neuroforamen. The needle at C4 was slightly withdrawn back after this view

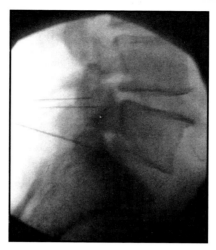

Fig. 37.23: Lateral view of the same patient, the probes are seen appropriately at C4 and C5. The needle tip should not be anymore anterior than as visualized on these views. Because of the shoulders, it is usually difficult to visualize the lower levels, but it usually can be done by coning the C-arm and using a slightly high output, but unfortunately with scanning the flouroscopic picture that view could not be reproduced

introduced. My choice is 20 Gz 100 to 150 mm long radiofrequency probe with a 5 mm active tip. The electrode is passed through the skin, subcutaneous tissues, and the muscles. A bony contact is made at the most lateral aspect of the concavity and, then the needle is slightly withdrawn and slipped anteriorly.

The patient is sedated very mildly during this procedure and is asked to report if they notice any pain going down the upper extremities.

The C7 medial branch occupies the lateral aspect of the superior articular process and can be found on the superior aspect of the medial end of the C7 transverse process. A probe is placed at the junction of the transverse process with superior articular process. Again, the C7 medial branch does not pass along the articular pillar so the angulation of the needle can be less caudally oriented as opposed to the medial branches at the higher levels.

The third occipital nerve has two branches, a deep branch and a superficial branch. To denervate the deep branch, the probe is placed along the concavity of the C3 articular pillar and sometimes the electrode has to be moved down to the upper half of the convexity of the C3-4 facet joints.

For the third occipital nerve, which is the superficial branch of the third medial branch, the radiofrequency probe is placed across the C2-3 facet joint. This is quite a large nerve with variable location. The first probe is placed along the middle of the C2-3 facet joints and then another denervation can be performed slightly superior and inferior to that. In the AP fluoroscopy view, the electrode is placed directly across the convexity of the joint.

Once the probes are appropriately placed; AP, oblique, and lateral fluoroscopy view is obtained. After confirming these three views, sensory stimulation is carried out at 50 Hertz. The patient usually notices a buzzing sensation in the back of the neck, between 0.1 to 0.5 volts at 50 Hertz; also sustained contraction of deep cervical muscles can be noted. Following this, motor stimulation is carried out at 2 Hertz. The motor testing is done three times the sensory threshold. The patient is carefully evaluated for any motor movement of the upper extremities suggesting nerve root stimulation. Once appropriate testing is done, 0.5 mL of 2% lidocaine is given through each needle and radiofrequency denervation is performed at 80 degrees Centigrade for 60 seconds.

Post-operative Recovery

The patient is given detailed instructions regarding the procedure and follow-up visit. The patient is monitored for any neurological deficits for 30 to 50 minutes in the recovery room and discharged home. The patients may have ataxia after this procedure which is usually self-limited if they focus in the distance to achieve balance.

Repetition

Radiofrequency of the medial branch can be repeated again. It does not permanently destroy the nerves. The cell bodies of the nerves remain intact and the nerve regenerates and the pain can reoccur. On an average, the patient can expect up to 350 to 400 days of complete pain relief and when the pain reoccurs, it is usually not as severe. Repeated radiofrequencies can be performed, but repeating within one year is not recommended.

REFERENCES

1. Shealy CN. The role of the spinal facets in back and sciatic pain. Headache 1974;14:101-4.
2. Shealy CN. Percutaneous radiofrequency denervation of spinal facets. J Neurosurg 1975;43:448-51.
3. Organ LW. Electrophysiologic principles of radiofrequency making. Appl Neurophysiol 1976;39:69-76.
4. Bogduk N, Wilson AS, Tynan W. The human lumbar dorsal rami. J Anat 1982;134:383-97.
5. Bogduk N. The innervation of lumbar spine. Spine 1983; 8:286-93.
6. Bogduk N. The lumbar mamillo-accessory ligament. Its anatomical and neurosurgical significance. Spine 1981;6:162-7.
7. Bogduk N. Macintosh J, Marsland A. Technical limitations to efficacy of radiofrequency neurotomy for spinal pain.
8. Lord SM, McDonald GJ, Bogduk N. Percutaneous radiofrequency neurotomy of the cervical medial branches. A validated treatment for cervical zygapophyseal joint pain. Neurosurgery Quarterly 1998;8:288-308.
10. Dreyfuss P, Halbrook B, Pauza K, Joshi A, McLarty J, Bogduk N. Efficacy and validity of radiofrequency neurotomy for chronic lumbar zygapophysial joint pain. Spine 2000;25:1270-77.

Thirty Eight

Intrathecal Implantable Devices

DK Baheti

INTRODUCTION

Intrathecal drug delivery system provides targeted delivery of medications and minimizes the side effects of morphine. Yaksh[1] documented the physiological basis of the pain relief due to intrathecal opoids as the modulation of inhibitory mechanism occurring at the spinal cord. The analgesic effect of intrathecal opioids are dose dependent and stereo specific. However opioid toxicity can be easily reversed with naloxone.

INDICATIONS

- Chronic pain due to malignancy
- Life expectancy is short
- Chronic pain due to spasticity
- Long lasting pain not relieved by conventional technique
- Failed back surgery syndrome
- Complex regional pain syndrome
- Post herpetic neuralgia.

CONTRAINDICATIONS

- Patient unable or unwilling to consent
- Known allergy to contrast
- Local infection
- Coagulopathy
- Pregnancy
- Concurrent use of anticoagulants
- Known systemic infection
- Coexisting disease producing significant CVS or respiratory compromise
- Immunosuppression.

DRUGS USED

Following drugs can be used alone or in combination:
- Local anesthetics
- Clonidine
- Opioid- morphine
- Baclofen.

Screening of Patient

Screening of the patient is mandatory before considering for intrathecal or epidural implantation of port or pump. Any interventional procedures should be done with informed consent. These procedures are preferably done in procedure room or in operation theater. The investigations such as complete blood count, bleeding time and clotting time are necessary. An intravenous line is secured. The monitoring of BP, SaO2, and ECG is mandatory. An antibiotic cover is necessary. The guidance of fluoroscopy is useful.

The opioid or other drug used for intrathecal or epidural screening should be preservative free.

The patient is hospitalized for few days during which time the infusion rate is gradually increased. The longer the trail time, the greater the likelihood of decreased placebo response. During trail period the monitoring of pain intensity, functional status, vital functions mainly respiration and other parameters, use of breakthrough medications is of prime importance.

Intrathecal Trial–It is done by doing either by lumbar puncture or implanting a temporary catheter. If intrathecal catheter is not available of to make the procedure cost effective one can use pediatric epidural catheter. The tunneling of catheter is done. The intrathecal dose of opioid is 1/300th of usual oral dose.

Epidural trial–It is done by putting epidural catheter. It performed similarly. The epidural daily dose of opioid is 1/30th of oral dose.

One time bolus–It is the method of choice for screening of these patients. The intrathecal dose is given and the monitoring of pain intensity, functional status, vital functions mainly respiration and other parameters, use of breakthrough medications is of prime importance for twenty four hours is adequate.

Side port Catheter-It is surgically implanted for trial. The advantage is adding an implantable infusion pump after successful trial. However the added risk of infection may be there.

The opioid (morphine) conversation dosage from other routes of administration to intrathecal is as follows:
- Intrathecal to epidural = 1:10
- Intrathecal to intravenous = 1:100
- Intrathecal to oral = 1:300

EQUIPMENT FOR INTRATHECAL IMPLANTATION

- Implantable intrathecal infusion pump
- Accessories- connecting tubes
- Implantable port with accessories
- Surgical trolly with appropriate instruments.

PROCEDURE

Before starting go through the details of the literature and video of the intrathecal implantation port or pump. Follow the instructions meticulously.

This procedure can be done either in local or general anesthesia. Follow the same procedure protocol done during screening trial of the drug. The pump, catheter tubings, connectors should be dipped in antibiotic solution for at least thirty minutes.

Step-1

Patient in lateral decubitus position identify the L3-4 space under fluoroscopy and do the lumbar puncture. Document the good flow of cerebrospinal fluid (Fig. 38.1). Clamp the catheter to avoid the unnecessary loss of CSF. Withdrawing of spinal needle will help to minimize the leakage.

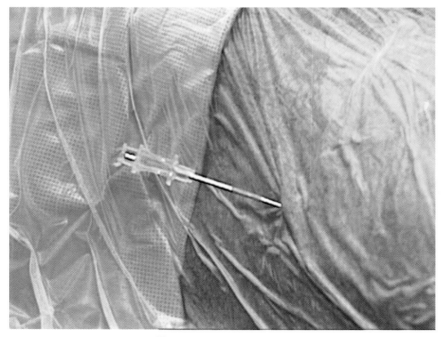

Fig. 38.1: Free flow of CSF

Step-2

Under local anesthesia make a paramedian incision for fixing and tunneling of the catheter.

Step-3

Under aseptic precautions and local anesthesia make 10 to 12 cm incision in lower quadrant of abdomen (Fig. 38.2). Fashion a subcutaneous pocket large enough to admit the implantable pump. The pocket should allow the placement of pump comfortably without struggle and prevent the rotation. As a guideline all four fingers should be easily admitted to metacarpophalengeal joints into the pocket.

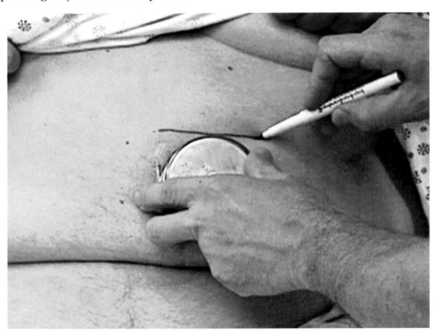

Fig. 38.2: Abdominal marking for implantable port

Undermine the upper side of incision about 2.5 cm or width of pump so wound can be closed without tension. A depth of 2.5 cm is ideal for telemetery. All bleeding points should be meticulously cauterized.

Step-4

Now, infiltrate, the track of tunneling with local anesthetic solution. Next, tunnel the catheter connecting intrathecal catheter to pump (Fig. 38.3). Pass the malleable tunneler device into the track of previously injected local anesthetic solution. Pass the catheter though tunneling device towards the pocket of lower quadrant of abdomen (Fig. 38.4). Confirm the free flow of CSF.

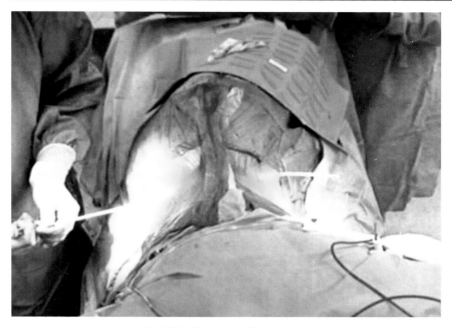

Fig. 38.3: Tunneling of the catheter

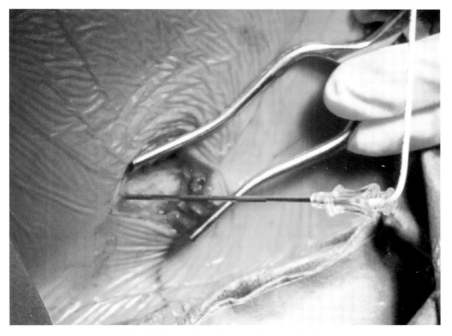

Fig. 38.4: Inserting the intrathecal catheter

Step-5

Fix the connection between the intrathecal catheter using, male to male tubing connector (Fig. 38.5). Tie this, joints with non 2-0 absorbable suture. Now take an anchoring suture with muscle fascia in figure of 8 fashion. This is to avoid migration of intrathecal catheter.

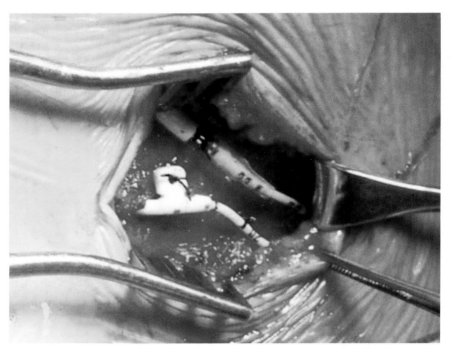

Fig. 38.5: Fixation of catheter in the lumbar area

Step-6

Aspirate any air in the programmable pump and fill the pump with the prescribed drug (Fig. 38.6).

Again check the free flow of CSF. Connect the extension catheter to the programmable implantable pump. Secure with 2-0 nonabsorbable suture tie. Place the programmable pump along with the catheter into the pocket at lower quadrant of abdomen. Confirm that there is no kinking of the extension catheter.

This is the diagrammatic representation of the pump *in situ* (Fig. 38.7).

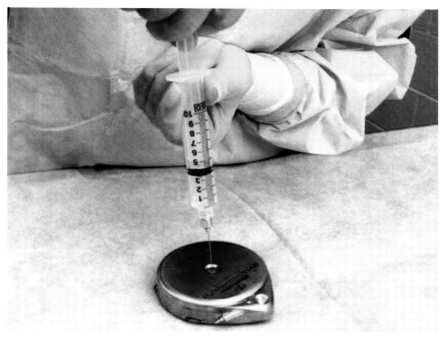

Fig. 38.6: Filling of the drug into the port

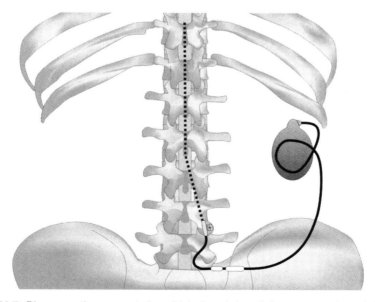

Fig. 38.7: Diagrammatic representation of intrathecal drug delivery system (pump) *in situ*

POST-PROCEDURE CHECK LIST

X-ray- Lumbo thoracic spine- Position of catheter.

COMPLICATIONS

- Surgical
  - Bleeding and hematoma
  - Epidural or intrathecal hemorrhage
  - Wound infection- site of implant or catheter
  - Meningitis.
- Implantable device related problems
  - Kinking of catheter: When residual volume of drug vary more than 20%
  - Solution- Fluroscopy or inject dye into the system (Before injecting dye remove the same volume of drug from system to avoid over dosage)
  - Volume discrepancy
  - Failure of self sealing septum
  - Battery failure
  - Pump motor failure
  - Failure of telemetery.

HELPFUL HINTS

A thorough conversation with patient and relatives regarding the procedure, side effects of opioid, possible complications is vital.

The length of screening trial is important.

REFFERENCE

1. Yaksh TL. Spinal opiate anaesthesia. Characteristics and principles of action. Pain 1981;11:293-346.

Section H

What's New in Interventional Pain Management?

Thirty Nine

Blunt Tip Needle

DK Baheti

INTRODUCTION

The iatrogenic complication during any interventional procedure are reported in literature such as in celiac plexus blocks are pneumothorax (two cases) by Brown[1]; partial lower extremity paralysis (One case) by Thomson et al[2]; temporary paraplegia (One case) by Baheti.[3] While performing lumbar sympathectomy Boas[4] reported 6% incidence of genitofemoral neuralgia, Cousins and associates[5] reported 35 patients with mild or severe neuralgia.

The other iatrogenic complications such as chylothorax, pleural effusion, renal injury and injury to veins also have been reported. The neurological complications include disestesias, paresis in lower extremities, paraplegia due to ischemia, spinal neurolytic injection, spasm of anterior spinal artery. P Raj et al[6] mentioned the complications such as backache, intravascular or subarachnoid injection, neuralgia, muscle spasm.

The role of tip of needle in above mentioned complications can not be ruled out.

The probable cause of above mentioned iatrogenic complications can be the use of sharp tip or short bevel needle, which may results in a puncture of an internal organ like vein, pleura, peritoneum and etc., and as mentioned above, these iatrogenic complications have been reported in the literature from time to time.

RECENT ADVANCES AND ITS IMPLICATIONS

The blunt tip needle (Fig. 39.1) recently introduced by Baheti DK[7] for these blocks (celiac plexus block and lumbar sympathectomy) may further reduce the incidence of iatrogenic complications such as injury to vessels, internal organ, peritoneum and pleura.

The new blunt tip needle is a 20-gauge 15 cm or 6"needle made up of stainless steel (locally made), which can be repeatedly autoclaved.

This needle is successfully used by author in more than 300 interventional pain management procedures which includes celiac plexus

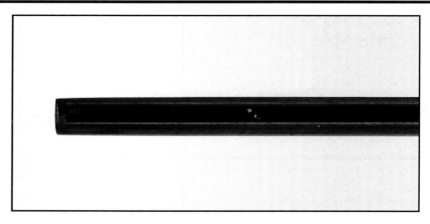

Fig. 39.1: Blunt tip needle

block, lumbar sympathectomy, and hypogastric plexus block and there is no incidence of injury to any vessel or viscera.

The author has also used 31/2″ needle for single shot epidural and transformational lumbar epidural successfully.

However it is found that blunt tip needle is not suitable for caudal epidural block as there is difficulty in puncturing of sacrococcygeal membrane.

The patent for the above needle is applied for.

REFERENCES

1. Brown DL, Bully CK. Quiel EC. Neurolytic celiac plexus block for pancreatic cancer pain. Anaesth Analg 1987;66: 869-73.
2. Thompson GE, Moore DC, Braidenbaugh LD. Abdominal pain and alcohol celiac plexus block. Anesth Analg 1977;56:1-5.
3. Baheti DK. Neurolytic coeliac plexus block (NCPB): A ten year review of 212 cases. Bombay Hospital Journal 2001;43(1).
4. Boas RA- Sympathetic blocks in clinical practice. In Stanton-Hicks M (Ed). International Anesthesia Clinics. Regional anesthesia: Advances in selected topics. Boston, Little Brown 1978;16(4).
5. Cousins MJ, Reeve TS, Glynn CJ, et al. Neurolytic sympathetic blockade: Duration of denervation and relief of rest pain. Anesth Intensive Care 1979;7:121-35.
6. P Prithviraj, et al. Celiac plexus block and neurolysis. Radiographic imaging for regional anesthesia and pain management. Churchill Livingston 2003;164-74.
7. Baheti DK. Use of new modified needle with blunt tip for neurolytic sympathetic block in abdominal malignancies- Abstracts, 11th World Congress on Pain: IASP, Press 2005;489-90.

Section I

Alternate Therapies

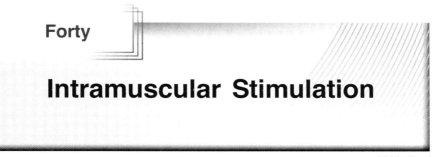

Forty

Intramuscular Stimulation

K Kothari

INTRODUCTION

Pain is the 2nd most common cause of physician visit after common cold. Musculoskeletal pain affects every individual at some or other point of his/her lifetime. Chronic myofascial pain or chronic pain that occurs in the musculoskeletal system without any cause is one of the most difficult conditions to diagnose and treat. Most of the available therapies usually give only temporary relief.

This technique is based on peripheral neuropathy mode.[2] This hypothesis believes that pain is the result of abnormal peripheral nerve function rather than a direct tissue injury.

History

In 1970 Dr Gunn noticed during examination of patients who had back pain for long period without signs of injury, had tenderness over muscle motor points in affected myotomes. He postulated that tender motor points are sensitive indicators of radicular involvement or irritation at the nerve root. Tender points differentiate a simple mechanical low-back strain, which usually heals quickly, from one that is slow to improve.[3] His study of patients with tennis elbow and shoulder pain showed that tender points at these points were secondary to cervical spondolysis and radiculopathy (i.e. neuropathy originating at the nerve root). Treating the neck, but not the elbow and shoulder was able to provide relief.[4,5]

Pathophysiology of Neuropathic Pain

Pain is a signal of tissue injury conveyed to the central nervous s tem via a healthy nervous system.

The definition of pain as given by the International Association for the Study of Pain, underscores this: "an unpleasant sensory and emotional experience associated with actual or potential tissue damage, or described by the patient in terms of such damage".[1]

The traditional model fails to explain many pain syndromes associated with damage to the peripheral nerve, or to the pathways coursing through the dorsal horn and spinal cord.

Why persistent pain occurs?

1. Inflammation do not subside despite of variety of treatment causing ongoing release of inflammatory mediators.
2. Psychological factors, e.g. somatosensory disorders, depression etc.
3. Nervous system malfunction–Myofacial pain is a neuropathic pain of the musculoskeletal system. These conditions are labelled according to their local sites like low-back pain, neck muscle spasm, facet joint pain, tennis elbow, lateral epicondylitis etc. The underlying mechanism is supposed to be supersensitivity of muscles[16] and muscle shortening.

Peripheral Mechanism in Neuropathic Pain

Sensitization can occur following tissue inflammation or damage to a peripheral nerve. Damage to the peripheral nerve is most commonly caused by spondolysis at root level (i.e. *radiculopathic* pain) when all fibers of the peripheral nerve can be damaged and can lead to any or all of the following effects: Muscle shortening, Autonomic (*complex regional pain syndrome*), trophic changes like dermatomal hair loss or weakening of tendons of muscle. These changes may be absent in early disease.

Initially term "pain following neuropathy"[6] was used but subsequently as it was realized that anterior and posterior rami are almost always involved, denoting radiculopathy (neuropathy at the nerve root), radiculopathic pain is more correct denomination.

Cannon and Rosenblueth's Law of Denervation

The normal physiology and integrity of all innervated structures are dependent on the arrival of nerve impulses via the intact nerve to provide a regulatory or trophic effect. When this flow (probably a combination of axoplasmic flow and electrical input) is blocked, innervated structures are deprived of the trophic factor, which is vital for the control and maintenance of cellular function. "Atrophic" structures become highly irritable and develop abnormal sensitivity or supersensitivity according to Cannon and Rosenblueth's Law of Denervation:[6]

When a unit is destroyed in a series of efferent neurons, an increased irritability to chemical agents develops in the isolated structure or structures, the effect being maximal in the part directly denervated.

All denervated structures develop super-sensitivity (including skeletal muscle, smooth muscle, spinal neurons, sympathetic ganglia, adrenal glands, sweat glands, and brain cells). Cannon and Rosenblueth's original work was based on total denervation and decentralization for super-sensitivity to develop, accordingly, they named the phenomenon denervation supersensitivity. But it is now known that physical interruption and total denervation are not necessary.

The supersensitive muscle cells can generate spontaneous electrical impulses that trigger false pain signals or provoke involuntary muscle activity[8] and supersensitive nerve fibers can become receptive to chemical transmitters at every point along their length instead of at their terminals only. Interconnecting pathways are possible between sensory and autonomic (vasomotor) nerves and may contribute to "reflex sympathetic dystrophy" or the "complex regional pain syndrome".

Spondolysis and Radiculopathy[1]

Of the innumerable causes of nerve damage, such as trauma, metabolic, degenerative, toxic, and other conditions, chronic attrition from spondylosis (the structural disintegration and morphologic alterations that occur in the intervertebral disc, with patho-anatomic changes in surrounding structures) is by far the most common.[6] The spinal nerve root is notably prone to injury from pressure, stretch, angulation, and friction. interestingly, neuropathy itself contributes to degenerative conditions.[7] Neuropathy degrades the quality of collagen, causing it to have fewer cross-links; it is therefore markedly frailer than normal collagen[9]. Radiculopathic pain syndromes should therefore be treated with some urgency to delay degeneration. Any degree of spondylosis, early or late can irritate and disturb function in the segmental nerve.

Muscle shortening is an early and common feature of radiculopathy. Painless, reversible, tight muscle knots can be felt in most patients even in young ones. Pain is not therefore a feature of radiculopathy unless nociceptive pathways are involved. Many neuropathies are pain free, such as sudomotor hyperactivity in hyperhidrosis, and muscle weakness in ventral root disease.

CENTRAL MECHANISMS IN NEUROPATHIC PAIN[1]

Interactions between peripheral and central mechanisms occur to produce post injury hypersensitivity and neuropathic pain. The spinal cord can modify or amplify incoming signals. Central sensitization, a state of hyperexcitability of the dorsal horn neuron, can occur after damage to a peripheral nerve or after low-frequency repetitive C fiber nociceptor input.[10]

Central sensitization results from:
- increased spontaneous activity of dorsal horn neurons[11,12]
- increased response to afferent input
- expansion of receptive field size– pain can spread to one or many segments up and down (by dispersion of the primary afferent input through propiospinal connections in adjacent layers 5 and 6 of the dorsal horn)
- reduction in threshold
- prolonged after discharges.

CLINICAL FEATURES

The history hardly guides pain physician towards diagnosis. Experience of examiner and his knowledge in segmental nerve supply myotomes are key to diagnosis.The physical signs of neuropathy are distinctive and one should always look for these as it is must for early diagnosis and treatment.

1. Allodynia: Muscles can be tender, especially over motor points. Autonomic vasoconstriction differentiates neuropathic pain from inflammatory pain, in neuropathic pain, affected parts are perceptibly colder.

2. Sudomotor activity: Excessive sweating may follow painful movements. The pilomotor reflex is often hyperactive and visible as "goosebumps" in affected dermatomes augmented by pressing upon a tender motor point, especially the upper trapezius.[1] There can be interaction between pain and autonomic phenomena. A stimulus such as chilling, which excites the pilomotor response can precipitate pain; vice versa, pressure upon a tender motor point can provoke the pilomotor and sudomotor reflexes.

   Trophedema: Increased permeability in blood vessels can lead to local subcutaneous tissue edema ("neurogenic" edema or "trophedema"). This can be confirmed by the peau d'orange effect (orange-peel skin), found over affected regions by "skin rolling", that is, by squeezing an area of skin and subcutaneous tissue. In trophedema, the skin is tight and wrinkles absent; subcutaneous tissue consistency is firmer; and the Matchstick test may be positive.[12] Trophedema is non-pitting to digital pressure, but when a blunt instrument such as the end of a matchstick is used, the clear-cut indentation is produced and persists for many minutes matchstick test). This simple test for neuropathy is more sensitive than electromyography.

   Trophic changes such as dermatomal hair loss may also accompany neuropathy.[1]

3. Trophic: Skin and nails can be affected, and there may be hair loss.

   Enthesopathy:[1] Tendinous attachments to bone are often thickened. Common sites are insertion of semispinalis capitis at the occiput, longissimus capitis at the mastoid process, deltoid insertion, common extensor origin at lateral epicondyle of elbow, origin of erector spinae.

4. Motor: Muscle shortening is a fundamental feature of musculoskeletal pain syndromes and of all the structures that develop supersensitivity, the most widespread and significant is striated muscle. Signs in muscle are therefore most relevant and consistent.

   Muscle shortening may be palpated as ropey bands in muscle. Focal areas of tenderness and pain in contractures are often referred to as "trigger points". Tender points can be found throughout the involved myotome. Muscle shortening causes a large variety of pain syndromes by its pulling effect on various structures.

Because the significant changes are primarily in muscle, *Knowledge of the segmental nerve supply to muscles is a clue to diagnosis.*

Even when symptoms appear to be in joints or tendons, it is changes in muscle that are most consistent increased muscle tone, tenderness over motor points, taut and tender, palpable contracture bands, and resultant restricted joint range.

During examination, each and every constituent muscle must be palpated and its condition noted. Palpation requires detailed knowledge of anatomy, and the skill to palpate comes only with practice.

Moreover, because many paraspinal muscles are compound (e.g. the longissimus) and extend throughout most of the length of the vertebral column, the entire spine must be examined even when symptoms are localized to one region

DIAGNOSIS

As already discussed history and lab tests give little assistant to the diagnosis, apart from above mentioned clinical features, some features that indicate neuropathic pain are:

- Pain when there is no ongoing tissue-damaging process
- Delay in onset after precipitating injury. (It generally takes 5 days for supersensitivity to develop)
- Dysesthesias - unpleasant "burning or searing" sensations, or "deep, aching" pain: which is more common than dysesthetic pain in musculo-skeletal pain syndromes
- Pain felt in a region of sensory deficit
- Neuralgic pain; paroxysmal brief "shooting or stabbing" pain
- Loss of joint range or pain caused by the mechanical effects of muscle shortening
- Abnormal bowel function (e.g. "irritable bowel syndrome")
- Increased vasoconstriction and hyperhidrosis
- "Causalgic pain"; "reflex sympathetic dystrophy" or "complex regional pain syndrome".[13]
  Laboratory and radiologic findings are generally not helpful.

Thermography reveals decreased skin temperature in affected dermatomes and this can be an indication of neuropathy, but does not necessarily signify pain.

TREATMENT

To treat myofacial radiculopathic pain is challenge. There are various options available to the interventional pain physician.

1. Pharmacologic Management: Is difficult.
   1. *Adequate sleep:* It is proposed that sleep disturbance occurs from a variety of reasons. TCAs help promote restorative sleep and heighten the effects of the body's natural pain-killing substances (endorphins), and increases non-rapid eye movement (non-REM) stage 4 sleep.

Low levels of serotonin and norepinephrine are related to depression, muscle pain, and fatigue.

Administering TCAs such as amitriptyline helps correct these deficiencies. Recommended dosing (Amitryptyline) - 25 to 50 mg 2 to 3 hours before bedtime, allowing peak sedative effect with minimal carry-over effect. May increase dosing to 50 to 75 mg over the next weeks if needed for added control.

Benzodiazepines are a second alternative, but should be used cautiously at bedtime due to their tendency to stabilize the erratic brain waves that interfere with restorative sleep in patients with fibromyalgia.

2. *Treat fatigue and depression:* If no response with TCAs, consider adding selective serotonin reuptake inhibitor (fluoxetine) in the morning. Recommended dosing 20 mg every morning (QAM). This class of drugs works to block the re-uptake of serotonin, which in turn allows the body to utilize greater amounts of serotonin. Treat muscle spasms. Cyclobenzaprine or low dose benzodiazepines (clonazepam) are used to treat muscle spasms. See explanation above for pathophysiological effect of these medications. Cyclobenzaprine also modulates muscle tension at a supraspinal level. Dosing is 10 to 30 mg every day (QD) or, if greater dosing is needed, divide the doses, with the smaller dose in the morning and the larger dose in the evening

3. *Adequate pain control*
   - Non-steroidal anti-inflammatory agents – Aceclofenac, paracetamol, diclofenac sodium, ibuprofen are all used. Most of the time they do not work well for these chronic conditions.
   - Tramadol may work for few patients. Dosage – 25 to 50 mg tds. Can be used in combination of paracetamol.
   - Muscle relaxants like tizanidine, Thiocolchicoside (Myoril) etc. are useful in relieving the muscle spasm in acute injury but their effect in chronic myofacial pain is not clear.
   - Local application of various gel/ointments like diclofenac/capsaicin etc. can be used. They acts as counterirritants .
   - Alternative therapies like hot and cold fomentation, massage can be useful along with physical therapy.

PHYSICAL THERAPY TREATMENT PRINCIPLES

The goal in treatment is to desensitize supersensitivity[15] by restoring the flow of impulses in a peripheral nerve. When the flow of impulses is briefly blocked, any supersensitivity that develops will also be transient. But when contractures and shortened muscles are present, their release is usually necessary to restore joint range and relieve pain: typically, when the several most painful contracture bands in a muscle are released, relaxation of the entire muscle follows.

Acupuncture

- Needle entry in the tissue stimulates it and releases contracture.
- Intramuscular stimulation is based on neurophysiologic concepts. Traditional acupuncture which is based on ancient philosophy.
- Acupuncture is a word of Western origin, coined in the 16th century to describe the Chinese use of a needle to promote healing in certain diseases.

Varieties of Acupuncture

Classical or Traditional Acupuncture, which forms part of the total entity of Traditional Chinese Medicine (TCM) is widely employed in China. There are various alteration to the acupuncture across the world but I will not go into details and we will discuss about this novel technique known as Intra Muscular Stimulation (IMS).

Intra Muscular Stimulation (IMS)

- This technique is an innovation of Dr C Chan Gunn, MD from at The Institute for the Study and Treatment of Pain (iSTOP), Vancouver.
- IMS is a system of dry needling that is based on a radiculopathy model for chronic pain.
- IMS requires a medical examination and diagnosis. It treats specific anatomic entities selected according to physical signs.
- Anatomy and neurophysiology knowledge is the basis for this therapy.

Equipments

- Cleaning solutions
- The fine, flexible, acupuncture needle. They comes in various sizes – 25 mm, 40 mm, 50 mm, 75 mm

  For superficial muscles 25 mm needles is used, for deep placed muscles longer needles are used.

Indications

- Chronic neck pain - spondylosis
- Frozen shoulder
- Achilles tendonitis
- Bicipital tendonitis
- Bursitis, pre-patellar capsulitis
- Carpal tunnel syndrome
- Cervical fibrositis
- De Quervain's
- Facet joint pain syndrome
- Hallux valgus
- Juvenile kyphosis and scoliosis

- Low-back sprain
- Plantar fascitis
- Piriformis syndrome
- Rotator cuff syndrome
- Shin splints
- Tennis elbow
- Torticollis (acute).

Procedure

The skin is prepared using betadine and alcohol. Under strict aseptic precautions the needle entered in the affected muscles. Needle is inserted at regular distance throughout the tender muscle band (Fig. 40.1). To assist the insertion of needle plunger can be used.

How much Deep to Penetrate

It is the experience of the pain physician to decide how deep one must go. Care is taken to avoid injury to any major vessels or important organs like pleura.

The activated and sensitized nociceptors of muscles are so exquisitely tender that firm pressure applied to it gives rise to a flexion withdrawal reflex (jump sign) and in some cases the utterance of an expletive (shout sign). The optimum strength of dry needling at a myofacial trigger point site is the minimum necessary to abolish these two reactions.[14]

When the needle penetrates normal muscle, it meets with little resistance. When it penetrates a contracture, there is firm resistance, and the needle is grasped by the muscle. The patient feels a peculiar, cramping or grabbing sensation - the "Deqi response".

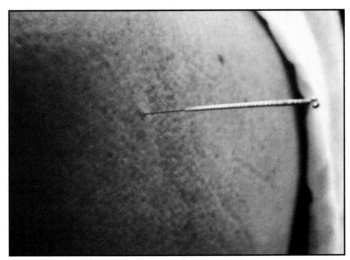

Fig. 40.1: Needle in position

When the needle enters fibrotic tissue, there is a grating sensation. Sometimes, the resistance of a fibrotic muscle is so intense that its hardness is mistaken for bone, and increased pressure on the needle may be required to force it in.

The Needle Grasp (Fig. 40.2)

When the needle penetrates a shortened muscle, it often provokes the muscle to fasciculate and release quickly – in seconds or minutes. A shortened muscle that is not quickly released, however, will invariably grasp the needle. The needle-grasp can be detected by the therapist when an attempt is made to withdraw the needle the grasp resists withdrawal. Leaving the grasped needle *in situ* (Fig. 40.3) for a further period (typically 10-30 minutes) can lead to the release of a persistent contracture.

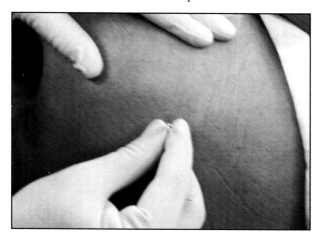

Fig. 40.2: Needle grasp

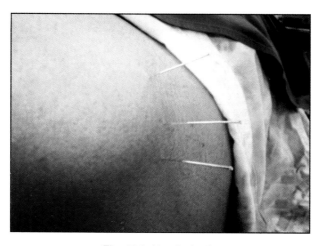

Fig. 40.3: Needle *in situ*

Failure of a correctly placed needle to induce needle-grasp signifies that spasm is not present and therefore not the cause of pain - in which case, the condition will not respond to this type of treatment.

When there are many muscles, each with many muscle bands or fasciculi requiring treatment, it may be convenient to hasten contracture-release by augmenting the intensity of stimulation. The traditional method is to twirl (rotate) the grasped needle - a motion that specifically stimulates proprioceptors. As an alternative to twirling the needle, heat (moxibustion) or electrical stimulation is sometimes used.

Needling can give magic response in many patients. Following needling, physical signs of peripheral neuropathy, such as muscle contracture ("spasm"), vasoconstriction and tenderness can disappear within seconds or minutes. (It is extremely satisfying to see these signs disappear before one's eyes). Other signs, like trophedema may diminish more gradually, sometimes even taking days to disappear, but ultimately, all signs vanish following successful treatment.

The needle as a powerful diagnostic and treatment tool: The fine, flexible, solid needle is more than a therapeutic tool, it is also a unique and powerful diagnostic instrument.

How does Twirling the Needle Work?

When a muscle is in spasm, muscle fibers cling to the needle, and twisting causes these fibers to wind around its shaft. This coiling of muscle fibers shortens their length, converting the twisting force into a linear force.

Unlike traction or manipulation, this stimulation is very precise and intense because the needle is precisely placed in a taut muscle band. The needle-twirling maneuver vigorously stimulates muscle proprioceptors and gives rise to a peculiar, subjective sensation known in TCM as the Deqi (formerly written as Teh Chi) phenomenon. This distinctive sensation is an extreme version of the muscle-ache felt in myofascial pain.

Twirling the grasped needle elicits the stretch or myotatic reflex. The reflex is activated by the muscle stretch and causes a contraction in that same muscle.

By stipulating the needle-grasp and the Deqi phenomenon as requirements for diagnosis and treatment, TCM has recognized the central role of muscle proprioceptors in chronic musculoskeletal (radiculopathic) pain.

In recurrent or chronic pain, fibrosis eventually becomes a major feature of the contracture; response to dry needle treatment is then much less dramatic and less effective. The extent of fibrosis present is not necessarily correlated with chronologic age: scarring can occur after injury or surgery, and many older individuals have sustained less wear and tear than younger ones who have subjected their musculature to repeated physical stress.

The treatment of extensive fibrotic contractures necessitates more frequent and extensive needling because release of the contracture is usually limited to the individual muscle bands needled. To relieve pain in such a muscle, it is necessary to needle all tender bands. It is rare to encounter a muscle that is totally fibrotic and cannot be released by accurate, vigorous needling.

Mechanism of Pain Relief in IMS

Ideally, stimulation should use the body's own bio-energy, which can be recruited in the form of the "current of injury".[1] First described by Galvani in 1797, this current is generated when tissue is injured, for example, following injection or dry needling techniques including acupuncture.

When the needle pierces muscle, it disrupts the cell membrane of individual muscle fibers, mechanically discharging a brief outburst of injury potentials referred to as 'insertional activity'.[1] Injury potentials delivered on needle insertion are able to relax a shortened muscle instantly or within minutes.

Needling also induces a sympatholytic effect that spreads throughout the body segment, releasing vasoconstriction.[1] Pain in muscles, tendons and joints caused by excessive muscle tension is eased when the shortened muscles are relaxed. Subjective improvement (which can sometimes occur within minutes) can be confirmed objectively; for example, as increase in joint range, or reduction of joint effusion. Endogenous opiates, now used to explain needling techniques, such as acupuncture, cannot account for all the observed effects.[1]

Unlike external forms of stimulation, stimulation from a needle lasts for several days until the miniature wounds heal.

Needling has another unique benefit unavailable to other forms of local therapy: It delivers to the injured area the platelet-derived growth factor (PDGF) which induces deoxyribonucleic acid (DNA) synthesis and stimulates collagen formation.[16] Body cells are normally exposed to a filtrate of plasmas (interstitial fluid) and would only see the platelet factor in the presence of injury, hemorrhage and blood coagulation.[1]

IMS differs from Traditional Acupuncture in that it:
- Requires a medical examination searching for early signs of radiculopathy
- Requires a knowledge of anatomy
- Requires a medical diagnosis that usually implicates spondylosis, uses neuroanatomic points that are found in a segmental pattern, instead of using traditional acupuncture points, determines the points to be treated according to physical signs. The effects of IMS appear very quickly and they can be used to monitor progress.

Post-procedure Care: This is day care procedure and patient is discharged from the hospital same day.

Injection of "Trigger-points": In recent years, the injection of "trigger points" has become widely used.

They differ considerably-

TRIGGER POINT	IMS
Localized phenomena - foci of hyper-irritable tissue	Super-sensitivity manifestations
Hollow traumatic needle with a bevel – may be harmful	Needle is pointed and solid almost atraumatic
Noxious source is not eliminated	Releases contractures – results in long-term relief
Injection of saline or local anesthetic, with or without steroids	No medication is injected
Serious side-effects due to steroid use may occur	No side effects due to injection

CONCLUSION

Musculoskeletal pain is radiculopathic pain involving segmental peripheral nerve supplying affected muscle. Diagnosis is mainly clinical. Diagnosis is by signs of neuropathy which are subtle but can be found if the clinician knows where to look, and what to look for.

Unfortunately, all external forms of physical stimulation are passive, and when application is halted, stimulation ceases.

Intramuscular stimulation is a great scientific technique which is based on anatomy (myotomes). The knowledge of myotomes is essential.

It requires minimal instruments (only thin solid flexible needles). Simple OPD technique and excellent results makes this technique very popular. It can be used in variety of conditions.

I will end this chapter with one massage – For many conditions IMS act as magic for the patients suffering from chronic musculoskeletal pain. Every pain physician must learn this technique to give patient a quality, cost effective and long lasting pain relief treatment.

REFERENCES

1. Loeser JD, et al. Gunn's intramuscular stimulation – The technique. Bonica's Management of Pain (3rd Edn).
2. Gunn CC, Neuropathic pain: A new theory for chronic pain of intrinsic origin. Annals of the Royal College of Physicians and Surgeons of Canada 1989;22(5): 327-30.
3. Gunn CC, Milbrandt WE. Tenderness at motor points—A diagnostic and prognostic aid for low back injury. Bone Joint Surg 1976;58A:815-25.
4. Gunn CC, Milbrandt WE. Tennis elbow and the cervical spine. On Mod Assoc 1978; 14:803-25.
5. Gunn CC, Milbrandt, WE. Tenderness at motor points: An aid in the diagnosis of pain in the shoulder referred from the cervical spine. JAOA 1977,77:196-212.
6. Gunn CC. "Prespondylosis" and some pain syndromes following denervation supersensitivity. Spine 1980;(5):185-92.
7. Cannon WB, Rosenblueth A. The supersensitivity of Denervated structures, a law of denervation. New York, MacMillan 1949.

8. Culp WJ, Ochoa J. Abnormal nerves and muscles as impulse generators. New York, Oxford University Press,1982.

9. Klein L, Dawson MM, Heiple KG. Turnover of collagen in the adult rat after denervation. Bone joint Surg 1977;59A: 1065-7.

10. Woolf CJ, Doubell TP. The pathophysiology of chronic pain increased sensitivity to low threshold AB-fiber inputs. Curr Opin Neurobiol 1994 ;4:525-34.

11. Woolf CJ, Thompson SWN. The induction and maintenance of central sensitization is dependent on N-methyl- D-aspartic acid receptor activation; Implications for the treatment of post-injury pain hypersensitivity states. Pain 1991;44:293-9.

12. Gunn CC, Milbrandt WE. Early and subtle signs in low back sprain. Spine 1978:3:267-81.

13. Kingerv WS. A critical review of controlled clinical trials for peripheral neuropathic pain and complex regional pain syndromes. Pain 1997;73:123-39

14. Baldry P. Superficial versus deep dry needling. Acupunct Med 2002;20 (2-3):78-81.

15. Munglani R, Hunt SP, Jones JG. The spinal cord and chronic pain. In: Kaufman L, Ginsburg R (Eds) Anaesthesia review. New York, Churchill Livingstone 1996; 12:53-76.

16. Thesleff S, Sellin LC. Denervation supersensitivity. Trends in NeuroSciences August 1980;122-6.

INDEX